"A true masterpiece that encourages readers to uncover the truth about their relationship to sex. The premise is that we can only heal our sexual issues if we look at the shadow side of sex squarely in the eye. This remarkable work does exactly that, covering everything from pornography to sexual abuse trauma. But then—Julie takes us a leap year further. She shows us that by examining our sexual wounds, we can transform sex into a means for enlightenment. I fully recommend this evolutionary approach to sexual healing."

—Cyndi Dale, author of 27 bestselling books including *The Subtle Body* series and *Energetic Boundaries*

"In *Sex Up Your Life*, Julie Archambault has paved a new and exciting path back to our natural state of health, harmony and happiness through the most overlooked portal: good sex. Compassionate, deeply researched, and peppered with fascinating stories, this book is the reliable empowerment companion we've been missing. Read it, do the exercises and pass it on—the sexed up journey can transform us, and the world, in the most gratifying ways."

—Caia Hagel, co-author of *Girl Positive* and co-founding editor-in-chief of SOFA magazine

"A brilliant commentary on the dark side of sex, the sexually derived wounds we carry and sex as the most powerful tool to awakening. Julie Archambault has done her research and presents her work in a colorful and lively way, masterfully interwoven with the occasional trigger warning as she leaves no stone unturned."

—Catherine Mellon, online business coach for female entrepreneurs

"Sexuality and intimacy can be complicated, messy, beautiful and personal – all at the same time. In *Sex Up Your Life*, Julie Archambault adds an important and clear voice to the necessary conversations on sexuality in all its complex reality."

—Rachel Braun Scherl, author of #1 International Best-Seller *Orgasmic Leadership*

SEX UP YOUR LIFE

The Mind-Blowing Path to True Intimacy, Healing, and Hope

Julie Archambault

COCREATIVE

CoCreative Press
Vancouver, BC
Canada

www.cocreativesex.com

Copyright © 2020 by Julie Archambault
First Edition — 2020

Terry Wong for Cover Illustration.

Julie Archambault for Cartoons.

Some names have been changed to protect the identity of certain individuals in the book. Thank you for your discretion.

All rights reserved.

No part of this publication may be reproduced in any form, or by any means, electronic or mechanical, including photocopying, recording, or any information browsing, storage, or retrieval system, without permission in writing from the author.

ISBN
978-1-7770653-2-4   (Hardcover)
978-1-7770653-0-0   (Paperback)
978-1-7770653-1-7   (eBook)

1. SOC065000 SOCIAL SCIENCE / HUMAN SEXUALITY
2. HEA042000 HEALTH & FITNESS / SEXUALITY
3. OCC011000 BODY, MIND & SPIRIT / HEALING / GENERAL

GET YOUR BONUS: "SEX UP YOUR LIFE WORKBOOK"

Get the most out of this book by downloading The Sex Up Your Life Workbook. You will:

- Be prompted with questions for deeper reflection
- Access your own story and healing
- Document your progress throughout the book

For a free download of *The Sex Up Your Life* Workbook, sign up for it here:

www.cocreativesex.com/workbook

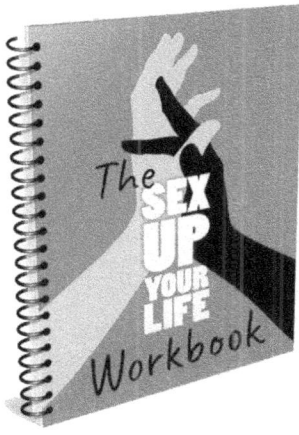
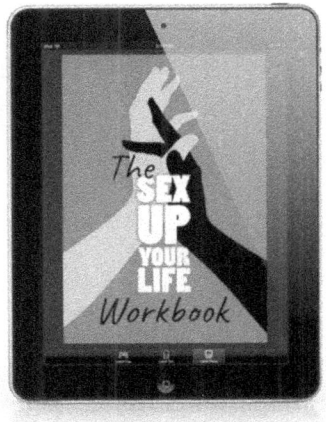

For Ogitchida Kwe, my loving warrior-sister

For the healing of sex everywhere

TABLE OF CONTENTS

Acknowledgement xi

Foreword xiii

The Owner's Manual: How to Use This Book 1

Introduction 7

PART 1 Sex on The Lower Continuum 15

Chapter 1: The Secret at the Bottom of the Barrel 17

Chapter 2: The Paradox of Sex Work 37

Chapter 3: Sex Under the Influence 73

Chapter 4: Porn-literate Meets Personal Development 93

Chapter 5: Decolonize Sex 117

    Section 1. Outgrow Power Dynamics 117

    Section 2. Beyond Orientation 136

    Section 3. Expand Gender 153

Chapter 6: Sexual Vampirism 161

PART 2 Sex On The Upper Continuum 183

The Clear Container 185

Chapter 7: Inhabit Your Body 191

Chapter 8: Time to Play 203

    Section 1. Expanding Play 205

    Section 2. Kinky Sex Can Heal You 213

Chapter 9: Remove the Armor 225

Chapter 10: Co-Creative Sex 235

Chapter 11: Conscious Practices 257

Chapter 12: The Threshold of Mastery 289

Accelerated Healing 307

About the Author 309

Helpful Links 311

References 315

Acknowledgments 325

ACKNOWLEDGEMENT

I am full of gratitude for all the amazing human beings who have contributed to this book by sharing countless hours of vulnerable and authentic stories with me: Devi Ward, Destin Gerek, Hasina Juma, Seani Love, Diane Hill, Maria Palumbo and many others that have done so while requesting to remain anonymous.

Thank you Baljit Rayat for seeing me and illuminating my gifts. Thank you for our countless conversations on sex, teaching me to access beyond the veils, and igniting my courage to take this topic on.

Thank you to all for infusing this book with your wisdom and experiences. Your courage to share your stories, struggles, and breakthroughs with sex, trailblaze a larger scope of possibilities for us all.

May this collected wisdom and knowledge shape a whole new level of understanding and possibility for sex in the world. For all.

May a new paradigm be born!

FOREWORD
by Shawn Bearman

Him: What do you like?
Me: I don't know. Let's try it. If I like it, we'll do it twice.
Him: You know you're not normal, right?
Me: What's normal?

We still live in a world where talking about sex is "not normal." This is no surprise, given how most of us were raised. There were clear rules, weren't there? There were certain things you were allowed to talk about and certain things that you simply did not speak about. SEX was definitely one of those things. That didn't mean we didn't talk about it at all… we did! But only with very specific people in our lives.

How did we learn anything then? That's right, it was a crap shoot. Fifty percent got lucky and our first experience with sex was not horrible. The other fifty percent, not so much. The point is that most of us were shooting in the dark, with no idea how to reach the other end of the tunnel to shed light on the subject and eventually visit Nirvana, Heaven, or whatever else you want to call the orgasm of all orgasms.

Along comes an incredible woman named Julie Archambault, author of *Sex Up Your Life*, who had the knowledge, the energy, and the balls to ask the important questions. What does it take to cause true intimacy, healing, and hope in the area of sex? Why is that even important? Here's why: whether you know it or not, people with healthy, active sex lives live longer. It's not rocket science. Sex is important. It releases the right hormones and body chemistries. It calms the mind, the body, and the emotions.

Now, if she had created just a regular book, that would be extraordinary on its own, but we get way more than that. We have a whole continuum to work through. The book is written through a collection of stories; people that have experienced the good, the bad, and the ugly of sex. We get to see how they dealt with it and experience the world of it through their eyes. Their stories are emotional, funny, sad, and fascinating. I love that you can follow where it works for you—it's like a choose-your-own-adventure book for sex! Who doesn't love those?

What I love about Julie is that when she was confused, she didn't just stay there. Unlike most of us, instead of swimming in the pool of confusion for life, she decided to go on a journey of discovery. What's the smartest way to learn? Start with what you know, find others that know more, and document everything. That's really what makes the journey you are about to go on so powerful: start with where you are and go on from there. This book is your opportunity to create a whole new paradigm in the area of sex, intimacy, and connection.

Go ye forth and SEX UP YOUR LIFE!

Shawn Bearman
The Coaches' Coach

THE OWNER'S MANUAL: HOW TO USE THIS BOOK

Throughout this book, we will be navigating the dynamics of sex on *The Continuum of Connection: From Destructive Disconnect to Blissful Connection*, as we head for "multilayered mastery." I created the Continuum of Connection to help us sort through all the complex dynamics in sex.

In the first part of the book—The Lower Continuum—we look at sex when it is a destructive force in our lives. This section deals with the different shadows that show up in sex and how they impact us. We take a courageous look at some of the uncomfortable aspects of sex and how people have healed from these difficult situations. Without tackling our shadow, how can we learn and improve?

In the second part of the book—The Upper Continuum—we take on sex when it becomes an ally to our wholeness; when it is actually building us. We take time to understand all the various elements that are needed on our path to multi-layered mastery! This is the path to deeper connection to self and partner while being a roadmap to blissful connection.

A heads up: I'm well aware that sex is a very triggering subject. For many, there is still a lot of pain and shame attached to sex. At times, I will give you a "heads up" if the content could be difficult for you.

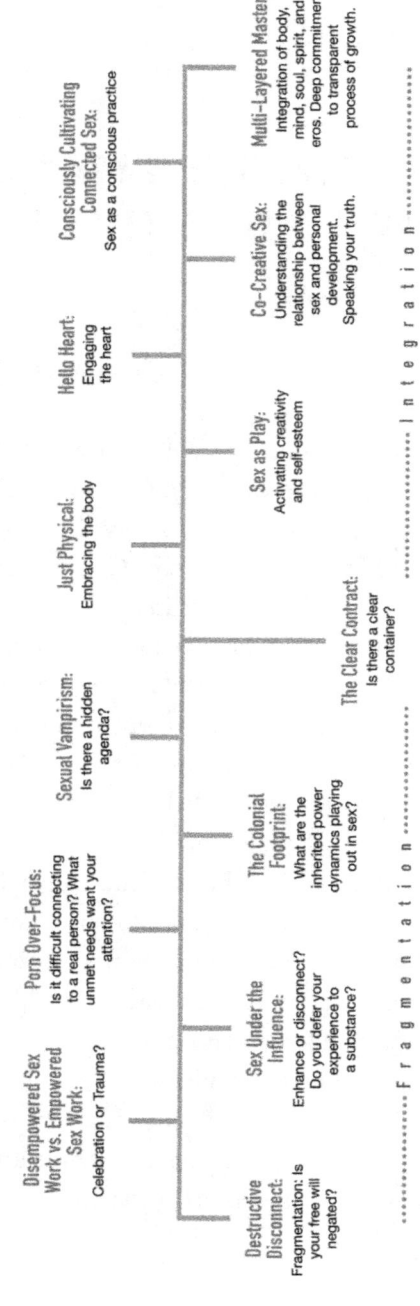

I designed this book to be a journey. Some of you will have already taken on this subject seriously and made some great strides in that department, while others may be waking up to this topic and to the struggles attached to it. There is something for everyone in this book.

You Have Options

If you are ready to jump in unapologetically and embrace the good, the bad, and the ugly, I suggest you simply read this book top to bottom to experience the buildup, the progression, and the unfolding of this mysterious force as it plays out in our lives and the wisdom it has to reveal to us.

If some of the more painful sides of sex upset you and would stop you from reading the book, PLEASE start with the UPPER CONTINUUM, Part 2 of the book. By doing this you get the benefit of engaging with the topic in a way that better meets your needs at this time. When you feel more equipped to take on the harsher sides of sex—the more confronting struggles—read the LOWER CONTINUUM, Part 1 of the book. This will allow you to bring serenity to all aspects of your life.

What is important here is that you respect where you are at and what you are ready to take on.

If you want to jump around, you can do that as well. You may want to start with the chapters that are most compelling to you and skip ahead, then scoot back. Each chapter stands on its own. But I'll still make my case: a profound picture is revealed when you behold the whole continuum—from destructive disconnect to multilayered connection.

Sex will mean a whole different thing to you once you've travelled through the entirety of the book. I invite you to take on the journey and to stick with it to the end.

No matter where you are standing, there is something for you in this book.

Please find it and start there.

Any strides you make, any leaps you make across this Continuum, are a triumph.

Chapter Design

Each chapter explores a theme on the Continuum of Connection and invites you into a real-life story that captures some of the dynamics at play there. Some stories have been shared by public figures that have accepted going public with their experiences. Others have consented to share their story anonymously with the hope that it would help someone else.

This book captures many interesting stories, but it can only contain so many. Every nanosecond a new story is born, a new dynamic experienced! This is a first attempt to glean a portrait, an overview, of the sexual struggles we face as a society. But rest assured, it is only the tip of the iceberg. This book, by its finite nature, can only attempt to offer a homeopathic dose of reality!

As you read, you may want to start writing down your own story with sex. Do it.

Each chapter has a section called "Soul Reverb" that is designed for you. It will help you access your experiences. Take time to answer those questions. You can download my workbook to help you with this task: https://www.cocreativesex.com/workbook.

Each chapter has affirmations to support you on your path of empowerment and integration. Come up with your own as well! Whatever is missing, you can create for yourself.

Get the most out of this book: be creative with it.

With love,

Julie

PANDORA'S BOX.

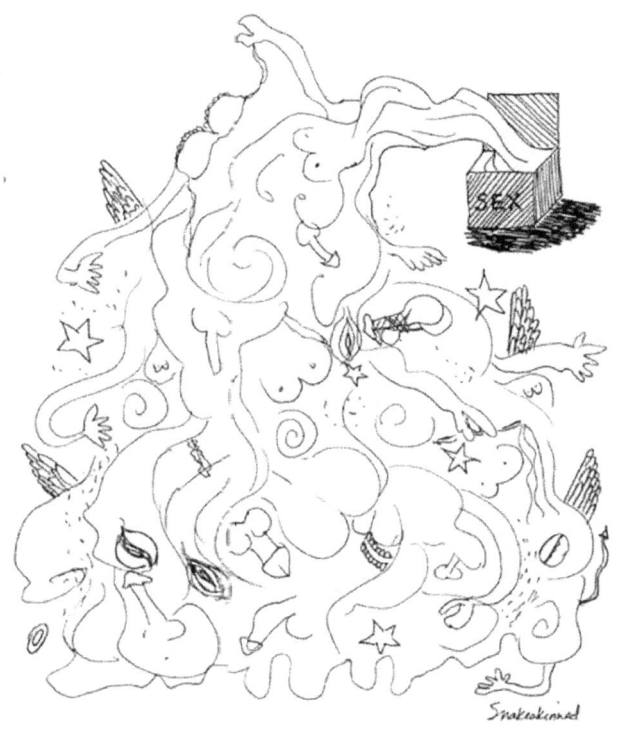

INTRODUCTION

This book started off with a simple question: "How is it that in one instance sex can be destructive, and in another, propel you to ultimate states of bliss?"

The short answer to this is: "Not all sex is created equal." I was trying to find a guiding principle that would help me sort through sex. "Connection" became my access. From this inquiry, I created the Continuum of Connection chart that you can find at the beginning of each chapter. Whatever I was discovering, I would test out with this question: "How connective is this sexual dynamic?" With this emerged Sex on the Continuum of Connection, from destructive disconnect to multilayered connection.

Each chapter deals with the nuances that emerge along this continuum. Sex can be quite complex—as we all know! Depending on the dynamics at play, you would be sliding across the continuum either gaining in meaningful connection or losing it. In the process of researching this, I interviewed many fascinating people about their sexual biographies, including cutting-edge sex educators devoting their lives to transforming sex in the world.

As I collected their stories, their struggles, their breakthroughs, significant revelations came into focus.

There are many wonderful books in circulation, bringing a wealth of knowledge to this intriguing force of nature. While some speak about sex in terms of biology, others construct themselves on challenging the status quo. Some are very practical handbooks, others more esoteric. I acknowledge that each approach gives us an angle to consider, a different vista from which to contemplate it. I am committed to creating yet another vista with the hope of giving an innovative access to this age-old mystery.

Coming from a background of holistic education, guiding students from grade 1 to grade 8, my mission was to nourish them in such a way that they would blossom to their fullest human potential. The commitment was to offer them a way to experience life and themselves in the most comprehensive way possible. This involved countless hours of learning, observing, adjusting, and a lot of finessing! This meant considering them not merely as brains to shape or fill, but as a full-fledged spiritual being, with a body, heart, mind, soul, and spirit. To behold this image of children was extremely helpful and broadened the scope of possibilities when designing their educational experiences. It gave us powerful access into important elements to address.

For instance, the "soul" needs powerful imagery and meaningful stories to be nourished. Stories allow for transformation, and I saw this on numerous occasions in the classroom. Problems suddenly resolved. Chaos dispersed into acute presence. Having this knowledge meant I had the keys to the kingdom! I will always remember the quality of listening on their faces when, in the oral tradition, I would recount collected mythologies and stories with strong archetypal characters, whether it be about Loki's conniving adventures, Alexander the Great's relentless expansion, or Cleopatra's poise and power. In these moments, the children would literally hang onto every word I would say. If I stopped a story halfway, there would be a collective cry in the classroom: "No! Keep going!" It was as if I was pulling away their plates too soon!

But the education, being the Waldorf Pedagogy, also considered developing all the senses through the arts: music to develop sensitivity to sound and tone, painting for an experience of color, movement to experience space and mindfulness. Sculpture for shape. Rhythmic repetition to strengthen the will and resolve. The whole faculty of teachers is devoted to this fine tuning of the human capacity. We were interested in the physical health, the "habit body" and "life forces" of the children, the igniting of their passions and feelings, and the awakening of their minds. We were astute in cultivating opportunities for mindfulness.

Why am I sharing this when the book is about sexuality? Because sexual energy is an important part in this picture that is often overlooked. To truly get sexuality and its impact on our lives, we must create the fullest, broadest picture of the human being and our potential.

When sexual energy awoke in my Grade 5 children, a class full of energetic and boisterous boys, I was peeling some of them off the ground and off the ceiling. It was somewhat of an emergency, and I wondered, how do I deal with this?! We tried a few things, but it left me feeling inadequate, unsure of the way to proceed. And when they were fourteen, they became curious and some boundaries were crossed amongst students—as they can with students at that age.

Regardless, it ignited this emergency siren in my soul. As a young woman, I'd experienced a similar crossing of my own boundaries, and since I hadn't fully addressed it, it woke up the mama bear in me who said, "This is not okay."

I showed up to class full of anger and reprimand, which in retrospect does not seem like the most astute pedagogical response. Essentially, I had not done the work of processing my own experiences, and that was getting in the way of my effectiveness. I'm sure some of the boys felt shamed by my response, and this book is a form of apology for handing over that shame, I did not know better. At the time, I had not done the work to be able to speak from a place of love instead of fear and hurt.

I came to see that if we don't take care of the issues lying dormant in our sexuality, it becomes very challenging to empower anyone else on the theme of sexuality. How can we transfer the awe and beauty of sexuality if we carry negative feelings about it? Being faced with sexual energy quickly brings us back to our unprocessed feelings that awaken fight, flight, or freeze! How do we educate in such a way that we don't merely equate sex to STIs, pregnancy, and risky behavior?

These issues were holding me back from being in a fulfilling relationship myself. At that point in my life, I was stuck. I knew I had to take this topic on to free myself. I started consulting with—and eventually learned myself—the healing modality of the Akashic Records. Every session would blow me away with insights into my life: for one, when and why I would go into fight, flight, or freeze. In terms of lost opportunities, this way of reacting had a major impact! I will touch on this later. This modality of healing would shed light on all those parts of my life that needed understanding. Every session would help me access more of who I was, and new possibilities started opening up. I was reclaiming my life, my voice, my power.

Then I started collecting stories of people's journeys with sex, which was the genesis for this book. How did sex play out in their life? What was going on for them, *for real*. I wanted to get the full picture. All this has led me to where I am today: guiding clients through healing journeys, both in online programs and individual mentorship series.

Clients now come to me for all kinds of reasons. They may be stuck outside relationships, in toxic sexuality/relationships, or they need help healing their sexual stories. Some are looking for break-throughs in a stagnating relationship, others simply lack comfort and ease with sexuality. I understood how deeply we need to talk about this topic, and what happens when we don't.

I also know that it is a taboo subject for countless people around the world. We are still collectively living out of our past experiences and traumas (big and small), our parental and family line's messaging about sex, our culture's context for sex. Add the dogmas from religion, history, and the colonial footprint, and we've got some hefty undertakings ahead of us.

Collectively, we need to dive deep into the heart of what beliefs and stories we are holding around sexuality to emancipate our-selves from them. By de-programming ourselves, we access our sovereignty. We experience alignment to our essence. We become powerful beings of creation.

This is no small, nor unimportant, task. As my friend and muse Devi Ward has said: "This is a revolution."

This is the journey: we will follow sex along this Continuum of Connection, from the gutter of human experiences to the heights of blissful expansion and see what powerful and helpful things reveal themselves about sex. As a "truth seeker," I hungered to hear about the real struggles rather than the mere superficial images given to the world and have honest and enlightening conversa-tions. So be prepared.

On that note, when something becomes too intense for you on this journey, skip ahead and come back later once you are ready to go deeper. Go for a walk, journal. Allow whatever is stuck to move. This can help you find your own path on the Continuum.

If you've experienced trauma, you may want to have help at arm's reach for support in processing the memories that surface.

Always remember that where there is reaction, there is a gift for you. It is pointing you directly in the direction of emancipation.

How do we fast track up this Continuum? How do we increase connection to self and to others? How do we fulfill our sexual potential and what does it take? This is the goal of the book.

My commitment is in helping us heal our relationship to sex in the world.

You will probably plot your sexual experiences across the continuum and from this get a better sense of what is going on for you and what direction you are headed. If we are honest, we are all here on earth to have an experience, which will be a unique path for each of us.

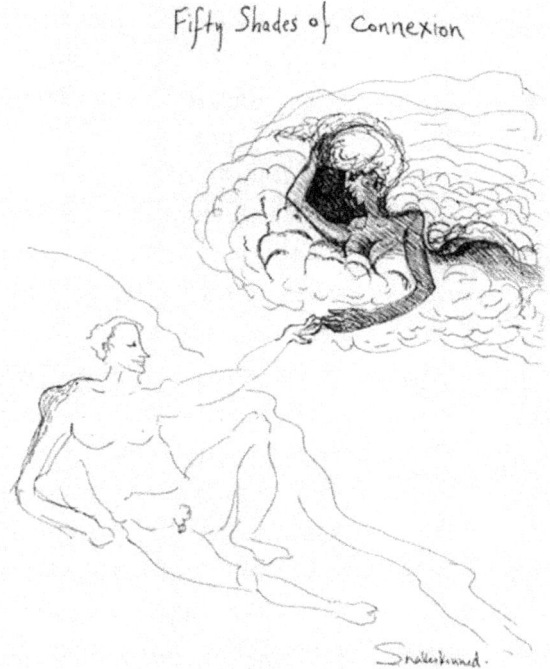

Fifty Shades of Connexion

GET ON THE FAST-TRACK

Before we proceed, imagine a beautiful porcelain vase filled with water and freshly cut flowers. Then watch someone, out of nowhere, pick it up and shatter it on the ground.

Let's take stock of what we see: shards of porcelain scattered on the ground. Water unfurling in all directions, container-less. Orphaned flowers laying distraught amidst the mess. Now, imagine collecting all those shards back into a pile in hopes of rebuilding the integrity of the vase, and mopping up the mess. Finding another container for the flowers to prevent premature wilting. Once the vase is glued back together, pouring water and restoring the salvaged flowers back to their rightful place.

This is the disarray of "fragmentation," and the careful piecing back into wholeness of "integration." This is what happens in sex: It can either fragment or integrate you. Such important processes beg to be understood to fully understand the power of sex. If you look at the diagram of Sex on the Continuum of Connection, you will notice the words fragmentation and integration.

Fragmentation means the process or state of breaking or being broken into small or separate parts. For the purpose of this book, it means experiences that break us down, alienate parts of our being, shut us down, block us from having access to them. These parts include our free will, our physical body, our creativity/playfulness, our sexuality, our power, our hearts, our voices. It involves the integrity of our mind, body, soul, and spirit.

Psychoanalysis defines integration as "The process by which a well-balanced psyche becomes whole as the developing ego organizes the id, and the state which results or which treatment seeks to create by countering the fragmenting effect of defence mechanisms." [1] For the purposes of this book, I will extend this process to restoring all the previously fragmented parts of our

---

[1] Lexico.com/en/definition/integration, powered by Oxford.

being alienated in response to physical, sexual, emotional, mental and spiritual pain.

If we jump into the realm of sex now, what would these two processes look like?

The first six chapters of this book, called the Lower Continuum, Part 1, address tales of disconnect, which can be understood as experiences of fragmentation where their wholeness is alienated into separate parts. We follow tales of people who have struggled and found ways to heal.

The subsequent chapters, the Upper Continuum, Part 2, explore tales of integration. Every story explores another layer of connection by accessing, first the foundation, the body, then the soul, which is enlivened through play, the power of confidence, the opening of the heart, the courage of self-expression, the investing of mindfulness in our actions, and ultimately, the accessing of higher spiritual experiences. The more you integrate and connect to yourself on all these planes, the more you become available for deeper connection. Simple, yet profound!

Imagine a xylophone with a full scale. Start playing a melody with the two bottom notes. Then add another note, then another, until you encompass the whole scale. The final melody will be quite different when you use the whole scale of possibilities. The melody will have a larger scope of expression, more nuances, and richness. This is the case with the varying levels of connection.

In "Sex Up Your Life," I am committed to helping you do this in a way that is of greatest service to you.

Hang on for the ride, collect all the symptoms of fragmentation to better see, and learn the art of integration to better create.

Ready?

PART 1.

SEX ON THE LOWER CONTINUUM

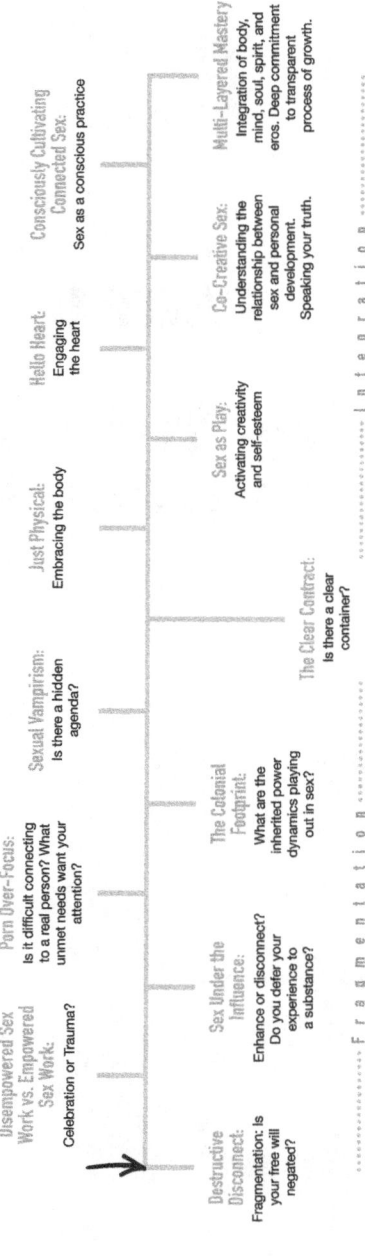

CHAPTER 1:

THE SECRET AT THE BOTTOM OF THE BARREL

"Everything in the world is about sex except sex. Sex is about power."

—Oscar Wilde

Poised at my wellness booth at the South by South West (SXSW) event in Austin, I greeted the participants intrigued by my topic—sex! They would scan my booth and then fixate on a large panel where I had glued *The Continuum of Connection.* "Here, take these stickers and plot your worst and best sexual experiences on the Continuum," I would urge them with a smile. Groups of friends would gather around the chart, read all the possibilities to each other, discuss, and then reach over the table to finalize their choice. Over the course of the weekend, the stickers cumulated on certain positions across the continuum, and some participants mused at the results.

"Wow," one visitor exclaimed, "that is sooo sad! Look at the number of people who have experienced sexual violation!"

I shook my head in unison, saying, "Indeed!" But really, is it that surprising? This is what the #MeToo movement sought to demonstrate. The truth is, sexual violation is a much too common experience.

In the U.S., one in three women and one in six men have experienced some form of sexual violence in their lifetime.[2]

The Centers for Disease Control's (CDC) National Intimate Partner and Sexual Violence Survey suggests that 44 percent of lesbians and 61 percent of bisexual women experience rape, physical violence, or stalking by an intimate partner, compared to 35 percent of heterosexual women. Twenty-six percent of gay men and 37 percent of bisexual men experience the same by an intimate partner, related to 29 percent of heterosexual men.[3]

The US Transgender Survey found that 47% of transgender people are sexually assaulted at some point in their lifetime.[4]

The numbers are staggering.

In this chapter you will:

- Discover violation in the realm of sex
- Experience Nancy's story of sexual violation and healing
- Identify loss of free will as fragmentation
- Understand the process of restoring self after violation
- Explore the various nuances of consent

---

[2] Smith, S. G., Chen, J., Basile, K. C., Gilbert, L. K., Merrick, M. T., Patel, N., ... Jain, A. (2017). The National Intimate Partner and Sexual Violence Survey (NISVS): 2010-2012 state report. Retrieved from the Centers for Disease Control and Prevention, National Center for Injury Prevention and Control: https://www.cdc.gov/violenceprevention/pdf/NISVS-StateReportBook.pdf

[3] The National Intimate Partner Survey, 2010, https://www.cdc.gov/violenceprevention/pdf/cdc_nisvs_victimization_final-a.pdf

[4] James, S. E., Herman, J. L., Rankin, S., Keisling, M., Mottet, L., & Anafi, M. (2016). The Report of the 2015 U.S. Transgender Survey. Washington, DC: National Center for Transgender Equality.https://www.transequality.org/sites/default/files/docs/USTS-Full-Report-FINAL.PDF

Before we start making sense of sexual violation in a broader way, let's dive into Nancy's story to anchor this into reality.

A heads up: There are some graphic descriptions in this story that may be disturbing. Keep your journal near and breathe through the difficult spots of the story. Reach out for support if the content is upsetting to you.

Nancy's Story—Piecing Yourself Back Together

Nancy signed up for a few sessions with me because high drama was a permanent staple in her household. It had decimated her marriage, was poisoning her relationship with her children, and had left her deeply dissatisfied with her life. She was deeply pained and hurt that her husband had left her and was dating a younger woman. Her teenage daughters would overtly taunt her with their highly sexualized attire, provocative activities on the web, and rebellious verbiage. Nancy's response to her attractive daughters was an utter desire to extinguish all outlandish behavior, shut out any sexual expression, and control the situation at all costs, even if it meant a storm in the house. She was the mother, after all, and she needed to set the rules and regulations in her own home. But all this drama was taking a toll on her health and her voice, which was essential to her career as a classically trained singer.

As we dug into her sessions, it became clear that her father's numerous sexual violations of her body as a child were essential in understanding the current drama in her life. Furthermore, as a teenager, a male friend had abused her on a camping trip, covering her mouth with his hand, like her father had done, while penetrating her non-consensually from behind. In addition, having a warped sense of boundaries as a teenager and young adult, she remembered finding herself in unsafe sexual situations, which on one occasion left her with herpes.

It became clear that, whether it be as a child hiding from her father under the dining room table or as a teenager escaping from that tent, sexuality was in no way a safe affair. Her strategy to maintain control and feel safe meant repressing her own sexual expression. She controlled her marriage to make sure her needs for safety were met. She controlled her children because she didn't want them to experience the sexual trauma she had. No one likes to be controlled.

When we started unpacking all this, Nancy was able to release some of these unconscious fears and programs that were playing out in her life. She released the fears that her daughters were at risk or that they wouldn't have the means to protect themselves. We retrieved the power of her voice by allowing her to speak her truth to her perpetrators via some role-playing scenarios. If she could use her voice, so could her daughters. This brought a certain serenity to Nancy. She also became aware of the grieving she had to do around not having fully experienced her own sexual and creative expression to its fullest maturity and lamented the costly impacts.

After a few sessions with her, I asked if I could interview her more formally and draw a much more complete portrait of her experiences. Her story is vast; she had worked many years on herself and could speak quite lucidly about her experiences and was, in fact, motivated by the hopes that her story could be helpful and healing to others.

The biggest challenge in Nancy's healing journey was actually remembering what had occurred to her, because for many years it was completely blocked out, and she didn't even remember that she had been sexually abused. Her father was a successful businessman with a strong, tyrant persona. He left Nancy's mom when Nancy was six, which meant that Nancy and her sister were to spend time at their dad's house alone with him. But by the time of this divorce, the sexual abuse had already started. The first memory Nancy had was of her and her sister, only four and two, in the bathtub and shower, being molested by him. Later they lived part-time at his house, which made the behavior occur more often. Nancy recalls deeply uncomfortable scenarios involving lying on the sofa and needing to smell his hands, with which he had probably masturbated. The memory of the smell still makes Nancy cringe today.

One of the more twisted sides of the sexual abuse was the pleasure the father derived in forcing his daughters to watch each other be molested by him. "I would have to watch my sister, and she would have to watch me, every night" Once, the father's girlfriend at the time had come home earlier than expected and walked in on him in the bathroom with his girls. Apparently, they broke up a little while later without any discussion about what had happened. Nancy also recalls that he would leave *Playboy* magazines open on pages with sexually explicit images. As a young girl, this would leave her feeling very uncomfortable. To wreak additional havoc, the girls didn't have a formal bedroom at his place; they would sleep on the sofas and didn't have a room for changing. This perpetuated a constant feeling of unsafety, which became her "normal."

For years of her life, she had no recollection of these memories, nor of many other things. She couldn't remember simple things about her childhood or teenage years. Her friends would reminisce, "Remember when we…," and she would be at a loss—she had no inkling of what they were talking about.

But most disturbing to her was when she was a young adult and went back to her family's time-share home in Mexico and found some of her childhood journals from when she was about fifteen. She remembers reading them from top to bottom and not recollecting a single thing. She had gone on a zip-line with a harness through the canopy, and she had been parasailing high up behind a boat that was pulling a parachute-like contraption.

"Like, how the hell is that possible that a fifteen-year-old girl goes parasailing behind a boat and doesn't remember that!? This is insane!" she said.

She went to find her sister in one of the rooms, and upon seeing the bed essentially went into shock: "I saw the bed and basically my entire body just lost it. I shat in my pants and peed all over the floor. I started screaming and crying. All of a sudden, I had the memory of being raped in that bed. It was from behind, my mouth was covered, and it had happened right there in that bed."

When she was reading about the parasail, of being so high in the sky, she would force herself to remember how that felt. And all she could think about was that for most of her life, this is exactly how she felt: flying, completely out of her body, hovering, looking down at her body from above. "I was just so out of my body. I could be that far up. It was so weird."

And so, by not being in her own body for most of her life, this also meant she had trouble remembering her life experiences. How could she? She wasn't actually "there"; she was flying outside her body. Called disassociation, this is a common experience when a person experiences trauma and doesn't feel safe—one leaves the body to survive the trauma and experiences amnesia. People feel detached from themselves and their emotions. They have a blurred sense of reality.

"That memory in Mexico was probably my biggest, worst memory to come to terms with, to believe and allow myself to believe that my father did that to me and deal with a huge argument with my sister because she was in denial and couldn't cope with it either," she said.

When this memory surfaced, Nancy underwent eight years of therapeutic sessions to work through the visions, the memories, and then the body memory. The surfacing pain was causing a lot of strife in all her relationships, including her marriage, and even in sorting through things with her sister. It ignited this raw anger within Nancy, and her sister just wanted to push her away, as if being re-traumatized herself from all their shared childhood scars and emotional upheavals.

In fact, as memories surfaced, Nancy would wake up angry even before the day had started. She often thought she'd better not go downstairs since she was so angry. At one point, she realized she had become addicted to anger, just like some people are addicted to alcohol. By this time, she was married with three children, and the seeds of chaos and drama were sown and thriving in the raucous family household.

After one therapy session, she came into her living room where the large dining room table from her childhood stood, the one that had been her hideout when she wasn't feeling safe. Suddenly, overtaken by an unleashed passion, she became obsessed with the idea that she had to get it out of her house. "To get that table outside of the house was a rebirthing. It was crazy; I needed that," she recounted. "I would go under this table, and I remember drawing under the top of it, hiding and hoping that I wouldn't have to do something with my dad."

After the incident in Mexico, she doesn't recall any other sexual abuse, but she does recall the moment she finally came back into her body. By this point, she was eighteen, had moved out two years prior to this, and had come to visit her father's cabin with her boyfriend. Seeing the boyfriend was quite a bit older than her, her father didn't want him to sleep in the same bedroom as her. "He started grabbing me and pushing me over the banister and stairs; it was a physical fight. He almost killed me. I don't know what happened, but I basically came into my body in that moment. I feel as if I woke up for the first time. Before, I mean, I was just surviving, but this time I was actually fighting him." It occurred as a life or death situation, and she suddenly felt this presence in her body, and this was new. "This is when he realized he kind of lost me, that I had a boyfriend, then later, a husband."

When she was eighteen, she started getting some of her memory back and started to witness when her "consciousness" would be outside her body. "I would walk home at night and I would be up at the top of the streetlight and I would start having these experiences as a regular occurrence. I would have to look into a mirror and try and bring myself back into my body instead of watching it from above."

Events started helping her wake up to her reality, including a boyfriend who had said to her that she herself was "abusive." "I was like, you are kidding me, right!? Like, I can't believe you are telling me that." The boyfriend had grown up with a counsellor as a mom and had the language to name what was going on. "I don't exactly remember what I would actually do to him, but I'm sure I turned into rage and I would say abusive things to him. Since I was a toddler, this way of acting was the norm." She also recognizes now, as she is finalizing the divorce papers with her husband, that she has existed in a state of perpetual chaos because that was her baseline. And what's more, that chaos has been very costly on her life, including on the people she cherishes the most, her children.

This is why she's had to dig deep into her story—so she could escape these perpetual cycles of violence and destruction. This involved taking on numerous healing sessions, including sessions of rebirthing and the twelve steps for children of alcoholic parents.

Nancy's story of healing is still ongoing. As her daughters continue to embody their sexuality, test out their own boundaries, and discover their sexual power, Nancy knows it is an invitation for her to grow and come to peace with her past. She also knows that her eldest daughter, who grew up in the era of Nancy's unleashed and unprocessed anger, has inherited a generous dosage of this unbridled anger herself, and is now flinging it right back at her mother. Furthermore, Nancy has a new partner in her life, which means more possibilities for growth ahead as challenges pop up in their relationship.

As our interview was coming to a close, Nancy told me, "Before, life was a constant stream of chaos, drama and screaming, and I didn't realize anything else was possible. Now, friends are noticing the change. I notice a change. I notice that peace and quiet are possible now. That there can be chaos, but that I don't need to be swallowed up by it." Another glimmer of hope: she just received a hefty grant to write a new music album. This may be an opportunity to turn some of these painful situations into art.

As for the effects of sexual abuse on someone's life, we can see with Nancy's story that the ramifications are far reaching, both in her own life and for those she loves. Here, we witness Nancy's powerful experience of being outside her body—the trauma response known as dissociation—where she has the sensation of floating over her own body. We also get to see what it means to feel fragmented—where you lose access to parts of yourself—and the subsequent striving and work of putting herself back together.

The Effects of Sexual Abuse

Research has documented some of the physical consequences of sexual abuse, which include genital injuries, sexually transmitted diseases, significantly greater difficulties with reproductive and sexual functions, and ultimately, post-traumatic stress disorder.[5] RAINN reports that, in the case of child sexual abuse, effects can be long-lasting and affect the victim's mental health.[6] Moreover, victims are more likely to experience the following mental health challenges: They are about four times more likely to develop

---

5 https://www.who.int/violence_injury_prevention/violence/global_campaign/en/chap6.pdf

6 Children and Teens: Statistics, RAINN. https://www.rainn.org/statistics/children-and-teens

symptoms of drug abuse, four times more likely to experience PTSD as adults, and about three times more likely to experience a major depressive episode as adults.

Within this context, it is quite obvious that sexual abuse is the exact antithesis of intimacy and connection.

From Nancy's story, we can appreciate how sexual violation can have many ramifications in our lives and stick to us over long periods of time. And if undealt with, it can be transferred onto the next generation. The impacts find their way into the most subtle and complex dynamics and patterns. But why?

Sexual energy is our creative life-force. Its nature is to move and circulate freely. Trauma is comparable to putting an unwanted dam in a river. The current is relentless in trying to move beyond it. This is why it will keep wreaking havoc in our lives until we take care of it. I will elaborate on unblocking our sexual energy in the Upper Continuum.

Let's Broaden the Picture

Sexual abuse includes all forms of non-consensual sexual violence done to an individual, including rape, sexual misconduct, molestation, and war-crime rapes. The American Psychological Association defines sexual abuse as "undesired sexual behavior by one person upon another. It is often perpetrated using force or by taking advantage of another."

As a society, the consensus is that sexual abuse is unacceptable. And yet, it still occurs across the globe. This form of sex is not about connection, but rather its antithesis—dominance and exerting power over another person.

So what defines this experience of sex? With violently disconnected sex, the individual is robbed of their "free will." They have no choice in the matter. As seen in Nancy's story, unwanted actions are done to them. Overriding "free will" is what shatters the vase on the ground. Considering that an essential part of our human dignity takes root in our individual "free will," something of our humanity gets fractured. The body no longer feels safe. One becomes fearful of future sexual encounters.

Trust and openness of heart are shaken. The victims are plagued with upset, anger, confusion, and fear. When free will is not respected, this starts the erosive process of fragmentation. In other words, we lose access to parts of ourselves that, until restored, no longer function as a whole. The mess of porcelain shards, running water, and broken stems lay disconnected across the floor.

Sex as a Weapon of War

What about sex as a weapon of war? You may, as I do, wonder how you can go from shooting and bombing people to sex!? Especially if you think of sex as an intimate experience. You wonder how one can get from combat boots and heavy artillery to something so personal. How can sex be brought into such a hostile environment? It is such a far cry from that exciting feeling of elation that comes with getting it on with your sweetheart. The short answer to this is: massive disconnection.

In the context of war, sex is intentionally and strategically made into a weapon to harm people. It has been used in various armed conflicts throughout the twentieth century, including Bosnia, Cambodia, Uganda, and Vietnam. To give a scale for this type of behavior, Rwanda has seen over a three-month period alone between 100,000 and 250,000 rapes.[7] Imagine the impact on the country.

According to the UN Action Against Sexual Violence in Conflict, "Rape committed during war is often intended to terrorize the population, break up families, destroy communities, and,

---

7 https://www.hrw.org/reports/1996/Rwanda.htm

in some instances, change the ethnic make-up of the next generation." When soldiers enter a village and rape girls and women, boys and men, they know the humiliation will last. The soldiers are showing them they have usurped their free will.

Sex here on the Continuum of Connection is intended to deeply harm the psyche of a village, town, or city. They are turning a penis into a weapon, to hurt, shame, dominate, and destroy. To contrast these experiences with the Upper Continuum, when sex tips into a form of integration, we discover that the penis, when coming from a healthy and loving place, becomes a remarkable tool for healing. But here on the Lower Continuum, it shows the disconnect between sexual organs and heart, a sure sign of fragmentation.

It would not be an understatement to say that these soldiers have some pain to process. Unresolved anger? Indoctrination? Powerlessness? They are certainly not coming from a place of love, nor wholeness.

Abuse Under the Radar

Now, let's go from this overt brandishing of one's sex as a public weapon of war to a more covert sexual abuse that is slyly concealed. Introducing Bill Cosby. He was accused of drugging and raping a whole slew of women and found guilty on three counts of aggravated indecent assault. When giving women the date-rape drug, he managed to tune out their consciousness, the very faculty needed to give consent. The damaging result was robbing them of sovereignty over their bodies, their desires, their decisions.

Now, entering more subtle grounds, let's look into a scenario where someone can, in fact, be conscious, but other forms of manipulation are used to undermine their sense of power.

With a long list of accusations attached to his name, Harvey Weinstein, the movie mogul, has become the poster boy for the

#MeToo movement. A statement from the New York Police Department said Mr. Weinstein "was arrested, processed and charged with rape, criminal sex act, sex abuse and sexual misconduct for incidents involving two separate women." Prosecutor Joan Illuzzi states that the former mogul "used his position, money and power to lure young women into situations where he was able to violate them sexually."

At the low end of the spectrum, the perpetrator is not tuned into the other person's body, nor their needs for safety, respect, and pleasure. These perpetrators are acting solely and violently to fulfill their own urges, without consideration of its impact on another person's physical body and psychological well-being.

Our Collective Purging

With the unfurling of the #MeToo campaign, harmful dynamics are now being magnified for society to see and appreciate the prevalence and nuances of this widespread problem. Whether it be the predatory Harvey Weinstein bullying actresses into fulfilling his sexual fantasies, the US gymnastic team's doctor Larry Nassar's abuse of position of authority with the young girls and women under his care, the experiences of sexual abuse by First Nations people at the hands of religious authorities as documented by the Truth and Reconciliation Commission in Canada, or common occurrences of non-consensual sexual acts on a date, and whether high profile or not, we are undergoing a long-overdue public purging of these abusive behaviors. Victims are finding a new confidence in speaking up.

BIG SISTER IS WATCHING.

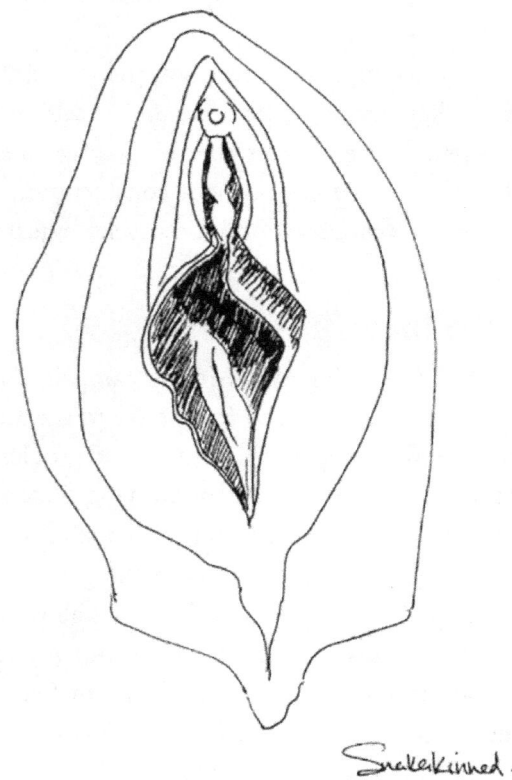

A proliferation of articles, shows, and social media threads have been dedicated to sorting through the cases that are surfacing. Everyone is grappling with the fine lines of what is acceptable and not acceptable, what is condemnable and what is condonable, and we are going through a serious process of clarification. And as a side note, the conversations get quite heated! The question remains: How do we come up with a new social contract that respects human dignity, for all with no exceptions?

Consent as Progress

Sarah Barmak, author of *Closer*, a book discussing the current emancipation of female sexuality and pleasure, has chimed in on the current conversation with an enlightening article on consent, published in *The Walrus* magazine. In it, she tackles the areas of ambiguity that often end up unspoken due to lack of clarity. She makes a helpful inventory that catapults consent into a whole new level of sophistication and awareness. She charts the evolving social mores as flagpoles that can guide our future social and sexual contracts. This is very helpful in navigating society out of this state of confusion and tacit "culture of sexual entitlement." It highlights how free will gets eroded and chipped away, while also giving clear signposts to reduce confusion!

These concepts will empower you on your path to freedom, bolstering our most reliable GPS: consciousness.

So here goes.

Coercion:

This occurs any time someone puts pressure on their sexual partner to have sex via manipulation, lies, insults, or continual insistence and arguments that wear down the partner. Barmark sums it up as being "verbally, emotionally, psychologically pressured into unwanted sexual conduct."

Compliance:

This happens when partners are not directly pressured into sex with overt actions or words, but regardless of their lack of interest or desire for sex at that moment they "comply" because based on past experiences they think it is the lesser of evils. If they opt out of sex, they might have to deal with another behavior that seems even more unpleasant, such as passive aggression, a bad mood, or on extreme ends, abuse. Sarah Barmark explains that people may not have agreed to having sex if they had felt more empowered to decline. This shows an important element: how empowerment and cultural conditioning play a major role. It also reveals that with more education and different cultural parameters, these dynamics can move out from the unspoken shadows.

Peek-a-boo from the Upper Continuum

Jumping ahead on the Continuum of Connection to forms of communication that allow for positive, integrative sex, the following serves to give you a better grasp of the fragmenting qualities *implicit in silence*, and to show via contrast what higher forms of consent actually look like.

Active Consent:

Barmark notes that the trend in society is towards "active consent," where you have a voluntary agreement that is reflected both with your choice of words and your body language. This is an important societal shift, whereby active consent is replacing "absence of a lack of consent"—putting the onus on the "active" partner *to get consent* rather than making the receiver the de facto "gatekeeper" who has to keep out unwanted behavior.

Sex Up Your Life

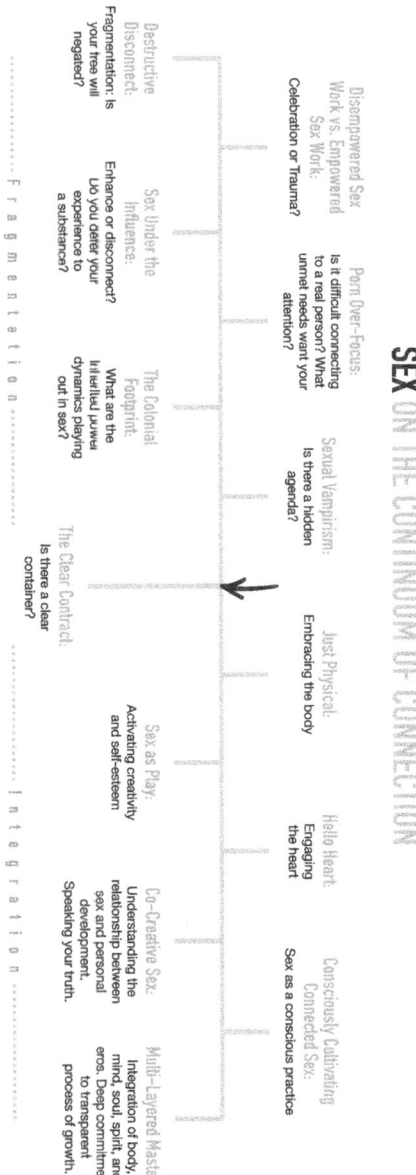

Enthusiastic Consent:

This is another level of consent that reflects the understanding that throughout a sexual activity, dynamics can shift, certain things may come up that you may not want to do or experience, or simply that your feelings may change, and there needs to be ongoing communication clearly showing consent and enthusiasm for sexual activity being performed and a space to hear a "no."

The core question to ask yourself in this shade of connection is: Has my free will been taken away from me? Is my free will under attack? Consistently worn down? Have I relinquished my free will? Or, can I say that I am an active participant here?

But there are some forms of sexual abuse that can't even be remedied by this new language around consent. Some situations are simply off limits, regardless of consent, due to an unformed adult ego. I am thinking of children, as we saw with Nancy's story, and perhaps some other cases of mental or emotional incapacitation.

In sex as violation, we can appreciate how disruptive and damaging sex can be if the whole human being is not taken into consideration.

Soul Reverb

Now that we have explored this difficult subject and appreciate Nancy's courageous journey of recovering physical, sexual, emotional, mental, and spiritual well-being after the harm has been done, let's take a moment for reflection.

I acknowledge you for taking on this difficult topic. If you have been hurt in this way, or know someone who has, I am sure you have many emotions surfacing right now.

Get a piece of paper, your workbook, or journal, and start by simply writing down anything that needs to find expression. Let it all come out. The more you get the poison out of your system, the better you will be. You may want to share your discoveries with a person of trust. You may decide to turn to professional help via a psychotherapist/coach to help sort through it all.

If you would like some guided questions, consider these.

1. Describe a time your sexual and body boundaries were not respected.
2. Can you define a time when sexuality felt off, creepy, or scary? How does this make you feel?
3. Does sexuality feel safe to you now? If not, describe why. If yes, take a moment to celebrate this!

Chapter Affirmations

- Sexuality is my life force and essence. It is safe to express my essence in the world. And it is possible, with help, to get through even the deepest forms of trauma.
- My sexuality is my creative power. The world benefits from my creative power. It is possible to find safe and empowering ways to express it.
- My body is my sacred temple. My voice allows me to set boundaries and have them respected. Everyone benefits from my healthy boundaries.

SEX ON THE CONTINUUM OF CONNECTION

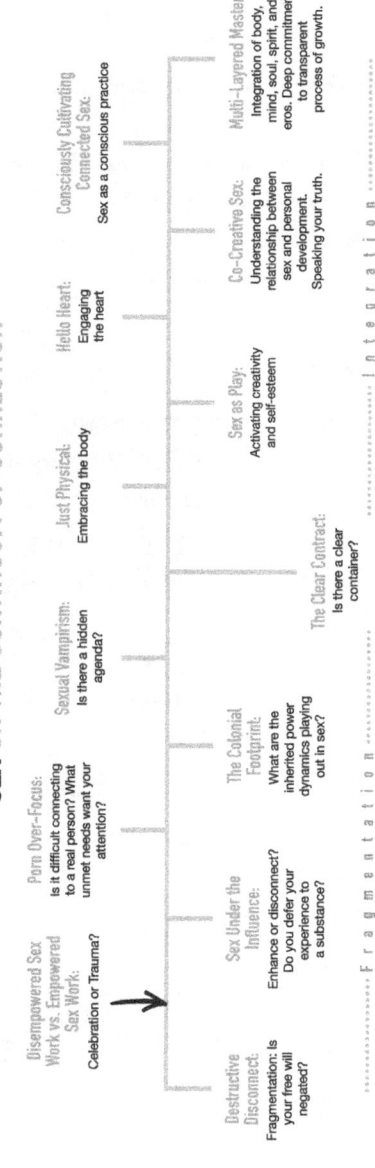

Destructive Disconnect: Fragmentation: Is your free will negated?

Disempowered Sex Work vs. Empowered Sex Work: Celebration or Trauma?

Sex Under the Influence: Enhance or disconnect? Do you defer your experience to a substance?

Porn Over-Focus: Is it difficult connecting to a real person? What unmet needs want your attention?

The Colonial Footprint: What are the inherited power dynamics playing out in sex?

Sexual Vampirism: Is there a hidden agenda?

Just Physical: Embracing the body

The Clear Contract: Is there a clear container?

Sex as Play: Activating creativity and self-esteem

Hello Heart: Engaging the heart

Co-Creative Sex: Understanding the relationship between sex and personal development. Speaking your truth.

Consciously Cultivating Connected Sex: Sex as a conscious practice

Multi-Layered Mastery: Integration of body, mind, soul, spirit, and eros. Deep commitment to transparent process of growth.

Fragmentation .... Integration

CHAPTER 2:

THE PARADOX OF SEX WORK

"Love conquers all things except poverty and toothache."
—Mae West

"I believe that sex is one of the most beautiful, natural, wholesome things that money can buy."
—Steve Martin

As we continue up the continuum, you've had a chance to reflect on your own sexual experiences and the areas where perhaps you felt violated as well. Chapter One may have stirred up many uncomfortable feelings: anger, dismay, sadness, perhaps shock. You may even notice how far you've come on your personal journey. This is no small feat. In this chapter, the intensity is not over just yet, but we are shifting gears: from difficult to empowered sex. Pour yourself a cup of tea, and let's dive into the fascinating world of sex work.

Now, you may say: "What does sex work have to do with me?" When you understand the impact intention has on the outcome of sex, what unconscious projections you behold, you'll understand that it is all relevant to uplifting your sex life.

The Paradox of Sex Work

In this chapter you will:

- Learn to distinguish empowered and disempowered sex work
- Explore how healthy boundaries are pivotal to the outcome of the experience
- Read Anne-Marie's story of disempowered sex work and Chatainya's story of empowered sex work.
- Learn the common physical, emotional, and psychological side effects of those who engage in disempowered sex work
- Consider how empowered sex work can enable sexual healing, empowerment, and social change.

Imagine for a moment a scenario where a sex worker goes to their child's parent-teacher evening at school and is asked what they do for a living. You can only imagine what must be going through their mind. *What will they think of me? What projections will be put on me? Will I be treated with less regard? How will my child be treated if they find out?* In some circles, the climate around sex work is changing, but if we scan the mainstream for its relationship to sex work, it is still a very uncomfortable subject for many.

I held my own judgements about what it means to be a sex worker and wanted to get to the bottom of this question of whether or not it could be empowering.

What is the reality of sex work? A lot has been communicated about the shadier side of the industry and trafficking. But is that the full picture? And if there is more, what can be said about the quality of connection possible with sex work?

As I interviewed various people in or close to the sex industry, an important distinction became clear. On the one hand, sex work could be experienced as a victimizing mechanism that brings sex workers down a disempowering spiral; on the other hand, when entered from a place of empowerment, sex work can be experienced as a place of healing, sexual expression, and celebration for all the parties involved.

For some sex workers, sexuality is their strong suit and cause for deep fulfillment. Some have trained in therapeutic approaches to help their clients overcome trauma. Sex work is of great service to people confused about their sexuality if they need to confirm their sexual preferences or orientation, or if sexual function appears out of order. The sex worker can help them sort this out in a private and helpful way.

It is no surprise that most of the time the topic of sex work triggers a high charge of emotions and strong views. You may yourself be skeptical that sex work can actually be a positive experience! People usually ideologically align themselves with one of the two camps: some are enthusiastically for sex work, and others vehemently against it. Some also view it as inherently sexist and a by-product of the patriarchal system.

Others view sex work as a means of sexual liberation and perfectly coherent with feminist discourse. In that view, a fully emancipated sex worker can freely choose to do what they want with their body, including their sexual expression. A sexually emancipated society is one whose values, infrastructures, and legal framework support sex workers to do this safely. In Germany, for instance, sex work has been legal since 1927 and the country has proper, state-run brothels. The workers are provided with health insurance, pay taxes, and receive social benefits like pensions.

The Empowered Sex Worker

Clearly, sex work is an extremely divisive issue. Yet, as I interviewed both empowered and disempowered sex workers, it helped me clarify what elements are needed for the sexual experience to be positive and connective. These are the very elements that allow sex to move through the Continuum of Connection and become a force of integration.

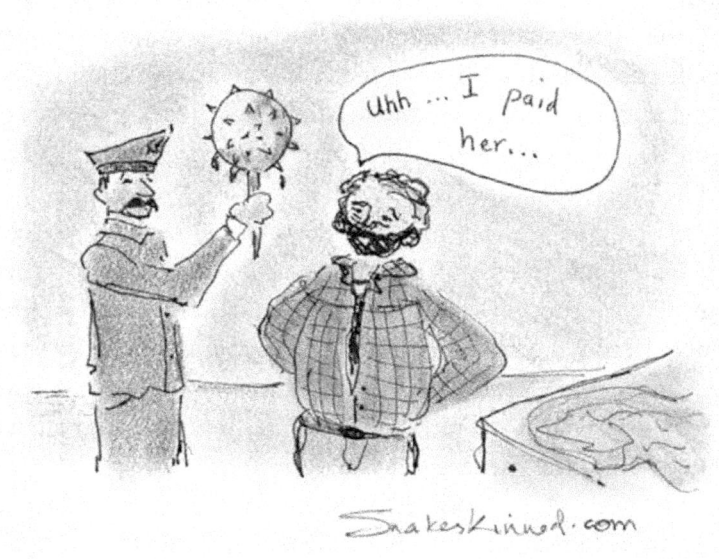

Someone who approaches sex work from an empowered stance has boundaries and knows how to establish a clear agreement. These people have defined what is acceptable and what is not for them, and they feel empowered to enforce this. They feel capable and actively speak up and educate their clients on the appropriate ways clients may engage with them. They have control over their schedule and their pay and have the freedom to choose the who and the how. They are aware of their needs and know how to make sure these needs are met. They also have a solid self-care practice.

In the most empowered situations, these criteria would also be backed by a favorable government, an informed legal framework, and an educated population to forge the safest context for their activity. Later in this chapter, you will read about Chaitanya's experience of empowered sex work, and in the Upper Continuum, you will read about Seani Love's mission and why he became London's joint winner of the 2015 Sex Worker of the Year award.

The Disempowered Sex Worker

Before we skip ahead, we must take a hard look at the mechanisms behind disempowering sex work if we are truly committed to transforming sex in the world. In a context of disempowered sex work, where vulnerable people are entwined in cycles of victimization and abuse, it deserves to be a neighbor on the continuum to "violently disconnected sex," especially in light of some common symptoms and impacts on their health.

But before we go any further, let's ground this into reality with Anne-Marie's story of disempowered sex.

Anne-Marie's Story—Clawing Out of Disempowered Sex Work

If you met Anne-Marie today, you couldn't imagine that she once was one of the ladies, as she says: "clawing herself out of the sex industry" for a better life. I met Anne-Marie while I was speaking at an event and she was on the expert panel. She is a tall, lush-looking woman, with long, wavy hair and a lovely tan.

When she spoke on the panel, there was authority and sensitivity woven into her alto voice. At the end of the event, she came to connect with me. "Hmmm, those ladies were really listening to you speak," she said, "it was so palpable." I had been speaking on the topic of Sex on the Continuum of Connection: from Violently Disconnected to Blissfully Connected Sex. I never would have imagined what she then said: "I was a disempowered sex worker. And I think your work could be really helpful to them."

To share your story as a disempowered sex worker is a very risky thing, especially if the wounds are still open. If the trauma is unprocessed, it becomes nearly impossible. If the shame and hurt are not released, you can't engage with the topic candidly. This is what was so inspiring about talking with Anne-Marie. She had been down the dark cave, and yet now she was back from the Underworld, and seriously kicking ass.

This is one powerful woman who earned it. This is one story that exemplifies the utter determination and power that can exist in one human being. Anne-Marie's story seemingly started off with financial ease. Her father worked in the oil industry, so they travelled the world to follow his work opportunities in Saudi Arabia, Russia, the Philippines and the U.K., amongst other places. She recalls a pretty comfortable life. Moving around like that gave her perspective on the world and gave her many unique childhood experiences. And yet, her young self could also detect the problems. Moving so much made it more difficult to establish real connections with friends, it was somewhat isolating, and she always seemed to stick out. She was different; very creative. She thought outside the box. Her striking beauty always brought attention to her, and not necessarily in a positive way.

There seemed to be a disconnect between her father and her that she could never manage to bridge, leaving her with feelings of neglect and of being unwanted. As she grew older, she saw that she didn't seem to benefit from the same quality of love that her seven-year-older sister received. These dynamics, coupled with watching how her father's long business trips away from the family and constant working, were tearing their family apart. Ultimately, it left Anne-Marie feeling quite bitter about him. She recognized that although her international childhood had been quite enriching and privileged, it had also left her with a significant amount of unsatisfied emotional needs.

At the age of twelve, Anne-Marie's mother left her father and moved from the Philippines back to New Jersey. From twelve to nineteen, Anne-Marie was barely in contact with her father, leaving the bitter taste of abandonment and resentment in her mouth, and the looping words "you were never there for me." By the age of twenty, her father passed away in the Philippines, his Filipino wife by his side, leaving Anne-Marie with many unanswered questions. The move back to New Jersey also proved to be a pivotal moment in Anne-Marie's story because her mother never took a penny from her father, and she put herself back into school.

It was a sudden drop from the more lavish lifestyle they had been living abroad; they had to start all over again from nothing. Some important associations started to be made at that point in Anne-Marie's young brain, such as: *Men equal money. Where there is no man, there is no money.* "There was a bridge happening in my brain," she said, "like my father is no longer there, and now we live in scarcity. So, there was definitely some of that going on at that age."

Just at that time, as she was an excellent athlete and student, one of the popular girls of the school took a dislike of her, and started spreading many rumours about her, unleashing some unfortunate bullying in her direction. This was obviously troubling for a young, grade-eight girl just growing into herself, already absorbing the multiple blows to their family safety net, not to mention the integration into a new school and a new life. "I was feeling pretty vulnerable to what people were saying to me and so that was definitely where a lot of the self-esteem and feelings of not belonging, really set in."

They were pushing on core wounds, such as abandonment and feelings of rejection, that had already been there from her childhood. And if this wasn't enough to cope with, Anne-Marie and her mother had to move again because the money was running out and they couldn't afford their home anymore.

They moved into a part of town where drugs and gang activity were rampant. Anne-Marie recalls being okay for a short while, but it was a slippery slope. "You know, put a vulnerable teenager with negative thinking patterns, self-esteem issues, and a sense that the world owes them something in an environment like that, I mean, it was pretty predictable." So by the time she was fifteen, she had dropped out of school, moved in with her drug-dealing boyfriend, was smoking up every day, and had held her first armed robbery for cash.

Anne-Marie recalls being out of control and just too much for her mother to handle anymore. Anne-Marie also notes that she always had a good heart, a lot of innocence, and wasn't somebody who wanted to hurt anyone; she was really just a sensitive person who had, by circumstances, created a hard exterior to protect herself. And yet, it was a time in her life she still feels lucky to have come out of alive. What sparked a change for her was when her boyfriend cheated on her. "I found out about it, and it was one of those startling moments in life that shifted me out of what was happening. I moved back home and recovered from that."

She recalls that at that point in her life she had bad acne and serious health issues. She had a whole slew of mental health concerns, spanning from anxiety and depression to suicidal thoughts. She recalls not having any friends and isolating herself. "I was feeling really shitty and just couldn't get out of bed in the morning."

When she was about nineteen, she decided to go see her childhood naturopath, and when she walked in, he said: "Oh, you are back!" She was feeling so sick, and was suffering from an autoimmune disease, with a litany of food allergies. He put her on an anti-inflammatory diet and the results were immediate. "What made it so easy to shift out of that lifestyle was that a lot of the cloudiness I was feeling in my mind, a lot of the anger and the rage, were actually triggered by my allergies. My allergies tend to trigger mental health issues for me. So, the way I was living, the drugs, the alcohol, the sugar, the dairy, were inflaming all these things in my body, so as soon as I changed my diet, in a matter of weeks, I couldn't recognize myself."

But another series of events emerged to crush her gains, pushing her into another spiraling depression. She found a waitressing job in a bar where a woman started reaching out to her. "Hey, you know, have you ever considered doing some modelling? You are such a pretty girl." Anne-Marie was pretty down and out and vulnerable at this point. She was plagued with self-defeating thoughts. The woman told her about someone living in New York who had women come and work for her. She said: "It's not like sex or anything; it's just like hanging out with these men."

Anne-Marie wasn't convinced but accepted that her information be passed on. In retrospect, Anne-Marie sees how clearly this woman was preying on her: going for a girl that was vulnerable, working in a bar, and clearly drinking. The other lady called herself a madame, but for someone who had no clue about the sex industry, this didn't mean anything to Anne-Marie. When the madame offered for her to come to New York for a weekend, it did not spell danger. "I have a private place; you can stay there, it's a beautiful condo. I'll give you two thousand dollars. Just come for the weekend, like, it's no big deal!" Anne-Marie enjoyed her weekend, and the money, and nothing was asked of her, so she thought, "God, this is nice! I could get used to this!"

When Anne-Marie inquired more about what this job entailed, the answer was basically, "You would be paid really well to spend time with successful men." From there, things started getting messy. She was invited a few more times and given the same generous sum of money to make her feel comfortable in the space. Eventually she started trusting the madame. The grooming process was slowly taking grip. It involved getting young women to let their guards down and then seizing control over them.

Soon the dynamic started shifting from generosity to "you owe me something." The madame would say: "Oh, I've helped you out so much, you know!" and start to make Anne-Marie feel bad. "Oh, will you come over this weekend? One of my girls can't see one of her regular clients, and I think you could do that! That would be great!" The madame slowly pulled her in, and finally, Anne-Marie agreed.

The first time was exhilarating, Anne-Marie remembers. It was pretty standard. "I mean, the guy comes in and puts the money down. You do it." Nonetheless, there was a lot of pain that came with it too. She would feel this inner dialogue go off in her head, saying, what am I doing!? "It was kinda of like waiting for it just to be over and needing the money to justify it to myself." In retrospect, there was also a lot of pain in being manipulated into this situation, without being told what was expected of her or given any real education about the industry or any of the terminology. "I went in there really blind, which is so not okay!" She recognizes that the industry attracts a lot of young girls just like her—still very naive and needing money. And yet, she says, "The situation was jeopardizing my safety, my health, my mindset, and my overall well-being because I just didn't know what was going on."

Then the looping syndrome sets in. Anne-Marie explains that this is a common experience for women who have been around the industry: "It's a very strange thing to say, but you almost become addicted to it because there is this monetary exchange and then you're also adored or appreciated or treated in a certain way, so it creates a lot of neurochemicals where, all of a sudden, you get this impression that your needs are being met. I mean, you are probably making more cash than you have ever made before, which brings this excitement piece, but it also comes with a numbing, jarring pain that I couldn't really distinguish at that point."

From an early age, sex had always been attached to a lot of shame and secrecy for Anne-Marie, which made the experience of sex feel disconnected. Within the context of the sex industry, these feelings were compounded, and sex started to feel merely transactional. Even outside the sex industry, Anne-Marie notes that it is a common experience for women to feel that sex is transactional. "There is this experience for women that this is 'just what you do'—you kind of please the man and it's, like, done." She recognizes that this is a very disempowered model for sex, and as she worked on the front lines there were a lot of these feelings going on for her where she was just waiting for it to be over and another layer of numbing added on.

While at the beginning it felt exhilarating, the further she got entrenched into it, the more disempowered, the more angry, the more hurt, she was. And the more addicted to the money she became. As she was working under the umbrella of the madame, there wasn't any space for choice, which meant she couldn't turn anyone away. "She was very controlling, and she was running us, so if you said no, or you did anything against the parameters she had established, she would just freak out." With sex work, Anne-Marie explains, there is choice, but then there is also an element of obligation. There is this odd paradox that sets in.

Women get talked into doing things, she says, and once the money is exchanged, "if the client does something weird, or shady, or suddenly you don't feel comfortable anymore, then it's like, do you give them their money back?" She explains that often that feeling of obligation overrides the woman's discomfort. "There is such an element of safety and trust when it comes to intimacy and sex, and when that's not created, and women have sex over and over again for money, there's almost this sense that sex becomes hardwired as an obligation, that it's performance-based, and it's not about pleasure."

She noticed that over time, she would be sitting in remorse, judgement, shame, and, of course, secrecy because she couldn't tell anybody, which brought on a lot of the darker and heavier debilitating emotions that got in the way of finding a new source of income. "I wouldn't be able to go out and create other money because I was steeping in all of these experiences that felt so shitty." She also noticed that she would spend her money faster, almost because she felt ashamed about the whole thing. "It became this loop where I'd have to keep going back and going back, you know." This went on for a while until she had a serious falling out with the madame and told her blankly to "go fuck herself!" She decided to go out working independently with a couple of friends, where they hoped to create a more empowering working environment for themselves.

But seeing she was struggling, being disempowered from the very start, she was still carrying all this baggage, all the accumulated scarring, that would weigh down on her experiences. "I was just reinforcing to myself all these stories, like that I'm broke, I will never be paid for what I love doing, I don't belong. It was becoming a fucking snowball, gathering momentum, and even just seeing it was challenging. We were all on a slippery slope. I was seeing all these women slip into drugs and get stuck in toxic situations, and I never felt like I belonged there." When Anne-Marie ran into acquaintances on the street, they wouldn't recognize her or feel like they knew her anymore. It was this form of dissociation that came with the double life. The other thing was that she didn't have a support system either, because it felt too shameful to talk about. When she finally spoke up about it to a friend, her friend was shaken up.

"It freaked me out to see my friend like that because I was like *oh my God, yeah, maybe this is really not okay.*" That is when she stepped back a little and started looking for other options. She found an escort company in New Jersey that was hiring somebody to work on their phone line to coordinate appointments. This gave her some space to start eating healthier again and feel better. It helped, of course, but she was used to making so much more money. Then the woman running the company started doing cocaine to lose weight. Since Anne-Marie already had addictive behaviors, it didn't take long before she started dabbling in it too.

"So within a couple of months, I was right back in there again, but the problem now was that I was working in my hometown, which really fucked with my head. I had never done that, and it felt way too close to home."

It propelled her into utter isolation. She would head downtown to blow hundreds of dollars in one shot. The proximity with the people she had grown up with while doing sex work did a serious job on her head. She couldn't maintain the separation, which meant the dissociation started to grow, and quickly spiralled out of control. She had always been a talented entrepreneur, and she knew that whatever she put her focus on, she could make into a success. The barrier had simply been some of those underlying stories she had collected over her life. "So, I just kind of got greedy. I was like, well, I'm so good at this, let me go and do this myself."

She put out an online ad looking for an investing partner to go into business with her. She had been in the industry for a few years now and knew how things worked and what the deal was. They could find an apartment and get their own sex-work services going. "I have no fucking clue what I was thinking. Nonetheless, toxic and addicted to cocaine, I would make myself believe that I was coming from this really empowered place. When, in fact, by this point, I was just so disempowered."

Some guy responded to her ad and seemed quite legit and just interested in finding some extra income sources. He found this swanky apartment and they launched the business. She found out later that his son was a drug dealer and the father had used his money for the apartment, which spelled trouble. By this point, Anne-Marie was doing cocaine all day, every day. "I started to completely unravel, so this was kind of the beginning of the end." The son started pressuring her to sell drugs to the girls working for her. And when the girls wouldn't show up for work, they started forcing Anne-Marie to work.

"They started threatening me: 'If you don't, you have to leave' and all those kinds of tactics." After about two months, she saw that this was really going south. At the time, she had met a guy that wasn't in the industry, but was still a toxic and unhealthy human being, and they latched onto each other. They both agreed that the situation she was in had to stop, so in the middle of the night they left for New York, and she had two grand in her pocket.

She was also very traumatized; she would wake up in the middle of the night sweating, with severe post-traumatic stress symptoms. She had gotten herself in very deep. "I felt like I couldn't control what was happening to me. I was completely unravelled emotionally, then physically, and my body was having some pretty significant reactions. I had panic attacks and I wanted to cut myself." She got a few phone calls from concerned people, connections from her criminal days, informing her to be careful because the drug dealer had put a hit on her head and was offering money to have her killed. She also worried about her mother, since he knew where her mother worked. Anne-Marie called a few people she knew to protect her mom. The man she was travelling with, her pseudo-boyfriend, started spending all her money on drugs, and was pressuring her to get back in the industry to generate some more money.

Many in the industry talk about the difficulty in leaving. "The women go to find the off-ramp, and it turns out to be really challenging because the money thing becomes an issue unless you have a lot of money saved up. The women say it's like you're trying to crawl your way out," she said. Add to this all the unprocessed trauma; she could be on a bus and if an older man simply looked at her, she would feel this violence ignite inside of her, like, "Don't you even dare look at me!" Anne-Marie explains: "I just felt so violated and, again, many women in the industry speak of this;

you feel like your body is not yours, as if you are an alien in your own body. It's a really strange feeling, and so there was a lot of reclamation that needed to happen." There had been so much dissociation, and she was now slowly starting to come back to herself and hear herself again.

When the money dried up, they hit rock bottom. Her so-called "boyfriend" was putting drugs up his nose every day and sleeping with all her friends. "I mean, he was a total mess, and I was trying to make a change here. So, I just said 'No. Get out of my life.'" She found a dingy hostel. "I just had enough for one night." She then got a job serving at a bar. She would go and work and make just enough to come back and pay for one more night. She kept doing that for two months. "I slept on this dirty cot and I don't think I slept a night. I was living off sandwiches and cigarettes."

She would scrounge up what little money she had left over so by the end of the two months, she had about six hundred dollars—just enough to sublet a room. "There were a lot of moments where I was like, oh fuck, it would just be so easy for me to go and find an ad online, because it's really easy to get into sex work. You call a number, and they'll send a driver. You disassociate for a few hours and you've got five hundred bucks in your pocket." Needless to say, it made it that much harder for her to hold on to the vision and conviction that regardless of having no money and barely having food to eat, this was it—no more. She no longer wanted to do this to herself. "There were some really rocky moments where I thought to myself, is this going to fucking work?"

For a while, it was just the next day and the next day and the next. "But luckily by that point, I had a pretty good sense of faith. I definitely had a sense of something greater than me, and I really feel like that's what got me through." When she finally moved into that room, this is when she really proved to herself that she could do it. She found a resource center which supported "prostitutes exiting the industry," and went there quite frequently to get support. Anne-Marie basically quit cocaine overnight but was still addicted to caffeine and ephedrine. "I've noticed that a lot of people that are disassociated use stimulants to simply show up for life on a daily basis."

Her life was starting to stabilize, but she still had many unaddressed post-traumatic stress symptoms. "I had a nicer home, I was healthy, I was getting back to a routine, I was working and felt better, but I also had a mountain of shame. It felt like I couldn't share this with anybody." She started dating a really nice guy and remembers breaking down at one point to tell him where she had come from and what her life had looked like just a year ago. It turned out he was supportive of her, and she told him she needed to put herself through recovery, saying, "I don't think I can manage how I'm feeling, and I need a break."

She got into the three-month recovery program and from this point went into the deeper, inner work, and pursued personal development to really clean up her life.

One of the reasons Anne-Marie agreed to share her story is because, as she says, "I think a lot of people believe, and even I believed this lie for a little while too, that there isn't a full life available after this kind of trauma, or that through a disempowering situation such as this you can't have the fullness of life back, but you can. I mean, I'm in a really beautiful relationship with my partner now, and I have a great sex life with him, and I have a really empowered relationship with my body, with men, with my work, and with money."

She says it was a long journey, and it took a long time to recover the safety around men. "That was a big piece for me." She recognized that for long periods of time she would wear masks and not let men have any kind of emotional relationship with her. "I would feel like my back would go up," she says, and she put up a strong masculine attitude as a defense mechanism to feel safe. Yet she would also burn out her adrenals from this hyper-masculine approach, workaholic and push-push success mentality. "I wanted to be successful, so I'd constantly push myself, but it burned me out."

Out of all this, Anne-Marie reflects: "The thing that is most fascinating to me, for some miraculous reason, is that I came out of all these situations still maintaining somewhat of the innocence about me. I still love people, regardless of all the turmoil and betrayal I experienced. I didn't let it completely harden me, and the more I healed from the trauma, the more I just let myself soften again. There was strength, there was grit, and intensity, but there was my heart, still there ready to trust. I've always been so grateful for that."

Anne-Marie's story is a testimony to the incredible power of the human spirit capable of overcoming adversity, even if it means crawling, or even clawing your way up the slippery and muddy slope of human misery. It's also a perfect illustration of a path of fragmentation, then recovery back to self.

So, What's Going On?

Anne-Marie's story does a good job illustrating many of the problematic dynamics involved in disempowered sex work. On the more extreme ends, sex work can involve enslavement and sex trafficking where individuals have been disenfranchised entirely of their free will, which is a direct parallel with the previous chapter. But sex work can also be a means to fulfill a desperate economic situation where sexual activity is a means to an end. When you have personal and economic disempowerment, sex work is in the realm of survival rather than an empowered choice. Although sex work has the guise of being a clear agreement, as we saw with Anne-Marie and the madame, in most cases, it is not.

Disempowered sex work is often entangled with other forms of pressures, such as grooming, trafficking, pimping, and various forms of coercive behavior. Research shows that many sex workers involved in disempowered sex work have been sexually abused, violated, or ill-treated earlier in their lives. This means that previous wounding and trauma is still playing out as a pattern in their current lives. If you never learned what healthy boundaries are while growing up, it will be difficult to know how to have them. Predators seek out vulnerable people because of this.

Until you have found the appropriate tools to reverse this pattern in your life, you will be grappling with porous boundaries, which puts you at a greater risk of re-victimization. It is not surprising that disempowered individuals participating in sex work end up with very similar symptoms to those of sexual assault victims. Furthermore, since it is repeated over a much longer period of time considering the nature of the job, the symptoms can be much more severe.

One of these shared symptoms involves post-traumatic stress disorder (PTSD). According to the Canadian Mental Health Association (CMHA), "Post-Traumatic Stress Disorder is a mental illness. It involves exposure to trauma involving death or the threat of death, serious injury, or sexual violence." It is prompted by something that is very frightening, overwhelming, and causes a lot of distress that the person was not anticipating and which they felt powerless to stop or change. The symptoms include: re-experiencing the traumatic event, nightmares, flashbacks, or recurring thoughts seemingly appearing out of thin air.

PTSD and Dissociation

People who suffer from PTSD may avoid situations that remind them of the traumatic event. The CMHA website explains that "PTSD can make people feel very nervous or 'on edge' all the time. Many feel startled very easily, have a hard time concentrating, feel irritable, or have problems sleeping well. They may often feel like something terrible is about to happen, even when they are safe. Some people feel very numb and detached. They may feel like things around them aren't real, feel disconnected from their body or thoughts, or have a hard time feeling emotions." The mental health organization notes that "alcohol or drugs can be a way to cope with PTSD."

A sure sign of trauma is indeed dissociation from one's own body. This involves fragmenting one's mind into parts to survive cruelty because the event is too difficult to process. PTSD is one of the ugly faces of fragmentation.

Disempowered sex workers can also experience a hyper-aroused autonomic nervous system. This means that the part of their nervous system that is responsible for the control of their unconscious bodily functions, such as their breathing, their heartbeat, and their digestive system, can suddenly flare up into jitteriness, hyper-alertness, and insomnia. They may also experience shortness of breath, muscle aches and pains, memory loss, vision problems, and stomach pains. Other symptoms include constipation and vaginal or anal pain.

Sex in these types of scenarios fragments your being, which also means the alienation of important parts of yourself—important elements that make you a thriving and whole human being. These symptoms are very powerful images of what happens with sex on the Lower Continuum. This is when sex becomes a destructive force.

Real Talk

In the "Garden of Truth: The Prostitution and Trafficking of Native Women in Minnesota"[8], the researchers document experiences of disempowered sex workers that can help us better grasp what this process of fragmentation could feel or look like. Here are some of the voices from the frontlines expressing how sex work has affected their lives.

---

8 http://www.prostitutionresearch.com/pdfs/Garden_of_Truth_Final_Project_WEB.pdf

One woman explains anonymously why she was taking drugs: "That is why I did a lot of drugs—to numb myself—so I didn't know what was going on and I could just leave my body."

Another woman explains how she would cope with the sex work: "If you're having sex with someone you don't want to, you leave."

One woman shares the impact of sex work on her psyche and the link to her childhood abuses: "There's times I space out because when I stop and think about reality, I break down, and can't handle it. I learned how to do that (dissociate) when I was a child being raped."

Within this context, it is not surprising that many of us can have a very poor esteem of sex work. It all sounds so very painful. Who would willingly chase after the discomforting reality of dissociation? Although a very authentic and disquieting reality, this is not the full picture. It is a journey in itself to shifts one's beliefs around sex work.

How about we transition out of these hardships and consider other possibilities. Let's follow Sylvia's surprising breakthrough in de-stigmatizing sex work for herself.

Sylvia's Story—A Past-Life with Sex Slavery

Sylvia remembered one past boyfriend referring to sex workers as "ball emptiers." This made her feel utterly insulted and triggered. She also remembered how angry she would feel when people lacked empathy when speaking about sex workers. She found herself collecting books on the sex industry and sex-worker biographies, curious about their lives and struggles. She found it peculiar that the subject was so intriguing to her.

Furthermore, she had found it baffling that a few of her close childhood friends had entered the sex industry in their late teens, regardless of their classic, private-school upbringing. Somehow, the sex work theme would surface in her life in the most peculiar ways.

One day, as her osteopath worked on her ankles, she felt startled by her therapist's comment. "Sylvia, there is such little movement in your ankles, it's as if you have metal leg cuffs on them!" The imagery was powerful. A few days later, as she was cleaning her room, everything became clear. She remembered as a child writing a surprising play about a chained woman who was made a sex slave for a sultan in the Middle East. Since Sylvia's upbringing included minimal exposure to such themes, it was a little odd that she would dream this scenario up out of thin air. Suddenly, she got this overwhelming sensation that it was a past life bleed-through: she had been a sex slave. She didn't quite know how to deal with this flood of new and "foreign" information, since she had grown up in a world where past lives were not a consideration.

Shortly after, she participated in a Quantum Energy Integration Program called Ka'nikonhriyohtshera: Fostering Emergence of the Good Mind, a healing lodge in Six Nations that is based in part on the WEL-Systems Institute's body of knowledge. During these sessions, all the participants, mostly but not limited to First Nations people from across Ontario, learn how to process deep-seated pain points, whether they are conscious of them or not. Sylvia decided to share with the group the surprising piece of information that she had recently come to understand. Diane Hill, the program director, didn't skip a beat. She asked her if she was ready to release all these cellular memories. Sylvia agreed. Diane then asked another participant to hold Sylvia's ankles while Diane felt guided to press a point on Sylvia's inner thighs. Bam.

The pain was excruciating. Sylvia screamed like there was no tomorrow and then sobs rolled in. Diane invited her to kick herself free from the strong male hands holding her ankles. She kicked herself out of the restrictive chains that somehow were still energetically attached to her ankles. This was very liberating for her. It was as if she was freeing herself from being chained to unhealthy situations in her present life, such as dynamics with her family and lovers. She no longer needed to endure their toxic behaviors. She no longer needed to passively be someone else's emotional punching bag or be used for quelling other people's sexual frustrations. She could simply walk away. Feeling like she had a choice was a profound change. She was now a free woman.

She also noticed that her perspectives opened up about sex work. Once she had freed herself of these past energetic imprints, sex work could escape the realm of victimhood. Sylvia went on to view sex work in a much more nuanced way. She no longer needed to project her baggage on other people's decisions and life choices.

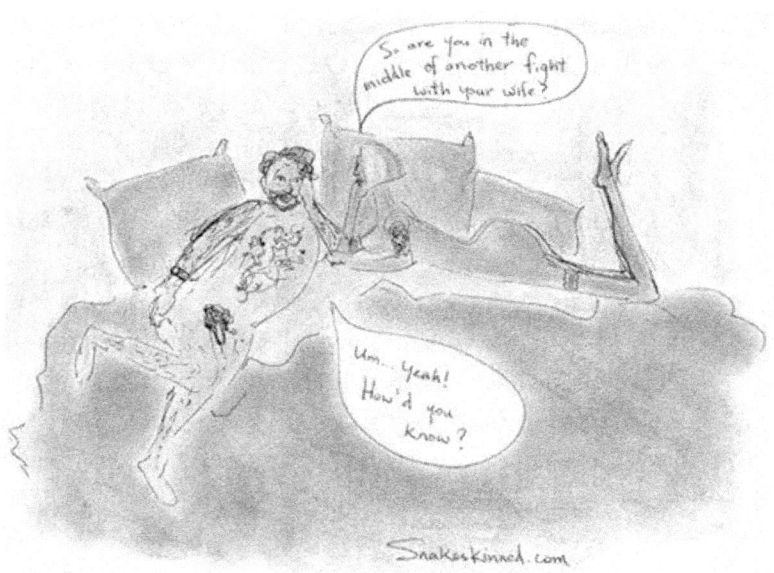

The Sex Worker's Purpose Today

Although we've just looked into stories that explore the shadow side of sex work, where free will is eroded, where the grips of disassociation and depletion take hold, this is not the full picture. In fact, it can be quite the opposite. When researching about empowered sex workers, some interesting and creative people started popping up on my radar. One was Zoë Ligon, a brilliant, millenial Detroit artist who transforms porn into edgy art while also owning Spectrum Boutique, a sex-positive, non-binary toy shop. She also amuses her Instagram followers with funny, provocative, and playful exposés about her yoni eggs, her art, her "girthy obsidian dildos," and her own sex work, earning her the title of "The Millennial Dr. Ruth" by *PAPER* magazine.

I also uncovered and started following London's 2015 Sex Worker of the Year, Seani Love. He shares his adventures in promoting Conscious Kink and the delicate art of consent, all while leaving behind trails of elated lady clients who line up to experience unexplored facets of their sexuality. In Chapter Eight, we will dive deeper into his story and how he uses Conscious Kink as a powerful path for healing and self-knowledge.

As I watched their work unfold, one thing suddenly dawned on me: empowered sex workers today have a very important role, especially when they combine it with a public persona and a desire to educate the population. They are the givers of permission. They are the ones that are leaning into sex, exploring and discovering all kinds of edges, finding the limitations and stretching out the collective possibilities. Many people have blocked sexual energy and secretly crave permission and encouragement for self-exploration. Having bold and relatable role models creates space for accepting sexual experiences as a legitimate part of our humanity.

Empowered sex workers are exploring and uncovering a much wider scope for sex in the world. If we consider all the negative spin that sex has received from all religions over long periods of history, all the shame and stigma that have been attached to sex by culture, education and socialization, empowered sex workers are actually on the front lines of freeing sex from its restricted and oppressed past. They are helping us create a sex-friendly landscape so people's sexual energy can begin to flow again and be experienced as natural, healthy, and empowering. By being so bold and open, they are helping people become comfortable with sex. Full stop.

A Shift Towards the Empowered Sex Worker

Although the old paradigm of "entitlement over women's bodies" is still present in our society, a new paradigm is already being created where reverence for people exists. Those who wish to be initiated into the art of sexuality and sexual pleasure can train under the guidance of highly skilled teachers and healers who have learned to create safe and sacred vessels to channel sexual energy in very positive and healing ways. When approached from this angle and within a quality container, healers provide an effective way for integrating those parts that need healing. Many of these educators are themselves empowered sex workers or former sex workers. They are leading us into this new paradigm as "sexperts."

Sex is a powerful and yet subtle energetic exchange. When that exchange is mindful, the potential for incredible transformation and healing is palpable. Empowered sex work requires appreciating what is involved in the energetic transaction in order to make a conscious decision.

Let's dive into Chaitanya's story as an empowered sex worker and hear what kinds of experiences she can create with her clients. It's pretty darn exciting.

Chaitanya's Story—Service, Impact, and Empowered Sex Work

Many years back, a friend who owned a sex shop said to Chaitanya: "You know, you would make a great dominatrix!" At the time, Chaitanya thought, "What the hell!? I didn't even know that existed!"

Being this all-mighty pixie-like blonde with what she calls a fiery Napoleon complex, she laughs and says, "You see, I compensate for my size. I fit into my twelve-year-old daughter's pants!"

Chaitanya does agree though with her friend's comment. "Well, you know, I am quite bossy, and I can be pretty controlling. I'm five feet tall, very strong, and trying to prove myself to the world!" Being an A-type, she was always the owner of the business, the manager of the organization, the teacher leading large classes. She even found herself pitching her business ideas on national TV. She had always been the one in control, with a strong masculine side to her personality. Yet everything about her life at that point in time was on a completely different track from sex work: she was a profoundly devout, meditating yogi clothed in white with every lock of hair wrapped in a turban. She could spend up to five hours a day in meditation and yogic practices. In fact, the path she followed was clear—she definitely was not to engage sexually with her students or clients.

She was on a path to awaken the full potential of her human awareness. She committed to refining and expanding that awareness to her unlimited Self. She actively worked to clear inner duality while creating the power to deeply listen and cultivate inner stillness. The goal: to prosper and deliver excellence in all that she does.

Yet her friend's comment also left a strong impression on her. Chaitanya was now curious to find out more, especially since she had moved to the city and was noticing how her women friends in sex work were doing so well financially. "They were very empowered. They had a lot of free time. They seemed really in control of what they were doing, how they were living their lives, and I was curious about it." She also was needing some extra cash and sought out some of the "sisters" doing the work to become a "sister-in-training." Chaitanya did a couple of sessions like this. They would offer tantra massage, which involves breathing exercises and sensual massage that ends with a hand release. The first two times, Chaitanya was a little nervous, as she had never done a hand job in front of anyone else. Fortunately, her partner took care of that. The lead sister told her how the session would go, and all Chaitanya had to do was observe and be present when giving the massage.

So, it was a very safe space for her. "The gentleman knew he was not to touch me, and the boundaries were very clear." Her trainer told her where to advertise and allowed her to listen in to a few conversations she had with gentlemen to learn the vetting process. She learned how to quickly establish authority with her clients. From the first conversation, she would clarify how the sessions worked and how to go about the "donation." In Canada, it's not illegal for a sex worker to offer services, but it is illegal to pay for sex, it's called a donation so it's not an actual financial transaction.

"I generally find that the older gentlemen would ask right up, 'so what is the donation?' because they are more educated about it." To find out that it was legal to offer sex work in Canada was comforting to Chaitanya; it was something that had concerned her before starting. "What if the police call and then show up at my house?" she wondered. "Then, I found out that it's not actually illegal for me. It's illegal for the gentleman." Part of Chaitanya's vetting process includes telling them straight off the bat, "I am not drinking. I am not doing drugs. I am not pimped out. I am a real person. I am an entrepreneur, and this is a conscious choice I am making." And this is a very important distinction to make. "I definitely always say that to them because I know there are people that are pimped out and I do not promote that in any way, and these men that are hiring people should be aware that they should not be taking that on either. So, I make sure to clarify that."

Being a single mom, she waited for her daughter to be away on a Thanksgiving getaway, and she thought that would be the perfect moment to test it out. "The house was empty, so I put up an ad and very quickly I came to understand that the men who respond are all different." Different ages. Different cultures. Different experiences in life. Different economic brackets. "I do charge more than, say, a woman that's selling on the street."

Chaitanya's biggest discovery was that these men are just like everyone else. "Maybe they need touch, maybe they need someone to listen to them, maybe they just need to feel seen. There are so many different reasons for them to come to me."

When they arrive in her studio, the first thing they do is have a shower. They come out with their towel fastened around them so they don't feel too vulnerable being straight-up naked in front of her. Then she sits with them at the edge of the bed and they talk about the clients' intentions for the session and what brought them. Chaitanya is dressed in a housecoat, under which she is wearing her bra and underwear. "So, I am contained in that way. Then I remove their towel and dry their back." She says to them, "Isn't it nice to have someone dry your back and take care of you?" In those moments, she often feels like the men are just like little boys.

"Then I take off my robe and we sit facing one another and we do breathing exercises. To get the sexual energy moving, you need sound, breath, and movement. And you know, in first-world cultures, we are holding on so tight that we don't even realize we are holding on. The breath and the sound are really helpful in letting go and relaxing into the present moment." During the breath work, Chaitanya and her client are gazing into one another's eyes.

She lets them know they can close their eyes if they feel uncomfortable. "It can be a very intense experience for someone to be really seen, because we don't generally have a lot of eye contact in our culture."

She notes that even just that experience in itself is quite powerful. Then, they'll inhale through the nose and exhale while sighing through the mouth to release a gentle "ha" sound. After several repetitions of this breath, Chaitanya will invite them to inhale through the nose and hold the breath in while squeezing their perineum, sex organs and navel center. In this way, the energy is pulled up the spine and when released, sending bursts of healing energy throughout the body.

The third breathing exercise Chaitanya does with them is a moving meditation. She gets a little bit closer to them and wraps her legs around them in the "Yab Yum" pose, which puts her sitting on him, and they hold each other and rock back and forth while breathing. While she inhales, he exhales, so it becomes a very powerful and dynamic experience. "Just doing that can lead to orgasmic experiences without penetration. So, I feel that this in itself is education. I will say to them sometimes: 'Isn't it amazing that we feel so orgasmic without actually having to physically have sex, without penetration, isn't this so powerful!?'"

The goal is to get that energy to move throughout all their body parts. Stagnation creates disease, physically, mentally, and emotionally. By guiding them through this meditative state, she points out how this is revitalizing their organs and how it brings peace to their mind. She gently brings their awareness to this process.

Then, she places her hand on his heart and invites him to place his hand on hers, while they gaze into one another's eyes. She brings in prayer, sometimes shamanism, sometimes essential oils, but essentially, she says, "We are just acknowledging the presence we are sharing. We are seeing one another. We are co-creating an experience. We are both human. We are both consensually choosing to be here. We acknowledge that I offer a service, that you are looking for a service, we agreed on an exchange and a donation that works for us. So, it's really clear."

In fact, it's so clear that Chaitanya has not had any problems. At worst, she has had to take a moment to educate her clients and steer them away from an entitled attitude around sex. "I gladly do this and tell them I am educating them for all the women in their life. So that they can know you can't just come in and expect to take me like that. It is always a mutually consensual experience." Chaitanya is very grateful for her solid boundaries, her authority, and her good fortune because she is well aware that this is not the case for all sex workers.

For Chaitanya, this work is very healing. For one, it helps her to balance out her masculine and feminine polarities. It allows her to experience what it is to be an empowered woman: "It means I have medicine inside of me." It also allows her to provide for her teenage daughter in a way that is very satisfying to her. She often tells the men that seek her services, "You probably thought you were coming for something, but the experience that you have had is so much more than that, and it may take a week to ten days before you begin to integrate what actually happened." This makes Chaitanya laugh. It can get pretty powerful and dynamic.

Some of the gentlemen that come and see her are going through major transitions in their lives. "I provide a very safe place for them to really let go, to express and be seen. It's a therapeutic and transformational experience." Chaitanya also coaches them. She combines counselling with this pure level of unconditional love while holding a space so they can really work out what's going on inside them. "I had a client who was going through a divorce. He had been married for twenty-five years. He just really needed someone to talk to, someone he could connect with. He had never been intimate with any woman other than his wife. For him, it was like I was his shaman goddess. He was so grateful."

Chaitanya believes that many times they are holding onto a lot of unexpressed emotions. For example, she talks about a man who had a woman's name tattooed on his body. When Chaitanya asked who she was, he told her it was his grandmother's name. She had passed away twenty-six years ago but he was still grieving her. He just couldn't let go of her. His grandmother had taken him away from an unhealthy family environment and raised him as her son. Through massage and essential oils, Chaitanya helped move the stagnant energy and he ended up sobbing. "I assured him: 'It's okay, your tears are welcome, your grandmother is here, she loves you.' He was on his belly and I just laid on top of him, naked, and held him, sort of like an orangutan mommy."

Once a gentle and kind man came in for a session. He had a girlfriend, but they weren't having sex. He loved his girlfriend, but their intimacy and sexuality had become dormant. He thought there was something wrong with him. Through the session, he got very stimulated and was able to ejaculate with the hand release. "He was, like, 'there is nothing wrong with me.' And I reflected back to him: 'there is nothing wrong with you.' He realized that day that he could allow himself to have pleasure." Chaitanya says that what she perceived before about this type of work and her actual experience are absolute polarities. What it comes down to is human connection. We all long to be loved, touched, and adored.

She says that having spent eighteen years practicing yoga really supports her in her sessions. "I would have a two-hour practice twice a day, well, because I was a wandering hippie! Yoga was my life!" She really learned to work with her kundalini energy, the primal life force stored at the base of the spine, so she knows how to bring that into a safe space for men. "You know, it is very helpful for the men. It is helpful to everyone, but 'big boys don't cry' takes away men's healthy processing of emotions. I provide them a place for that."

Chaitanya knows that her success comes from a strong grounding in self-care and healthy boundaries. To avoid depleting herself energetically and in order to not take on the men's energy, she has a series of self-care practices she does, including having an Epsom salt bath after her sessions. "They are really important so they can pull out all the negative energy and keep my energy field clean." She also adds essential oils such as thyme or melaleuca to the bath, which add to a deep sense of cleansing. Having a regular movement practice, as well as getting enough sleep and eating well, keep her strong and grounded in her body. She also loves to burn some sage to cleanse herself, the space, and her clients. She is very careful when scheduling. She avoids taking on too many sessions at a time. She knows that if she doesn't respect herself, everything will backfire on her.

"Once I went on a trip to Whistler and I had some time on my hands. So, I thought I'd put up an ad to make some extra cash, and I ended up getting so many responses that it was overwhelming." She lined up three one-and-a-half hour sessions and ran them like clockwork, telling herself, "At this time you arrive, by this time you will be in the shower, and by this time you will be dressed and on your way out." She says, "I had three sessions that night and the next day I woke up and had four more sessions. I had seven sessions in less than twenty-four hours, and I made twenty-two hundred dollars and I was like, 'holy shit,' and I was feeling good."

But three days later, she crashed and burned. "Literally the month of February, I made half of what I would have made because I gave so much and I took on so much. I didn't take the in-between times to take an Epsom bath, walk in nature, or do a meditation. And it's really important to do this to maintain balance in all things." She became acutely aware that when she over-gives, there will be a cost.

She clarifies that she never has sex just for money. "I did it one time, and I literally got sick right afterwards. I got an infection.

So, I know how sensitive I am, and I know that as soon as I do something out of integrity with myself, I create this 'dis-ease' in my body." This is why intercourse is always at her discretion. This also means that she has learned to navigate the conversations when the client would like some "extras" but she is not willing to go there. She does this by helping them refocus their attention on their process. She will say something like, "You know, this first session is all about you receiving, so even though you may have feelings, you have these thoughts, it's okay. You really want to focus on your breath so you can really feel what's going on in your body." She says this "helps them come back to themselves, instead of being in their heads thinking, or being stuck in their cocks!"

She is well aware that it's a delicate conversation with men and tries to navigate it in the most empowering way for them. One of her clients returned a few times. "He's just a nice guy, kind of like a brother vibe, and I don't do it with my brothers, and finally one day, he said, 'I just want to clarify how much it costs, and do you think there is going to be more interaction in the future?' and I said, "You know what, we're good where we are because for you, you also get counselling and coaching out of it, and you are really open to all of that, so if I were to take it to the sexual level then we're not going to have that space." And if ever a guy didn't accept it, she knows there are many other sex workers out there that would be a better fit for them. She doesn't worry too much about it.

She is also aware that men can fall in love with her. Whenever she feels the vibe, she makes it clear to them that this is her work. She is also mindful that she can be the one thinking, *oh my, is this the "one"?* It can be daunting at times when the chemistry is so orgasmic. In the business, they call it falling into the Cinderella-consciousness. One of the best pieces of advice a friend told her was, "Don't turn a good client into a bad boyfriend. Once they get sex for free, they will never pay for it again."

"Some of them adore me, worship me, love me, call me goddess. Others bring me gifts, like I said, they are so respectful! They know I am the boss, and I also receive so much out of these experiences."

And what about being a dominatrix? Well, it's something that is still on the radar. But Chaitanya wants to educate herself to see if it is actually a true fit. She also sees other things in her future. When her daughter is sustained and independent, Chaitanya has her own vision, which includes stages, speaking, and being more visible with her work and her message. Chaitanya has lots to share as an empowered sex worker holding a container of light and sacredness, both for herself and for her clients' embodiment and transformation.

What inspires me about this story is how sex in a solid and clear container can allow for people to heal and grow. Sex work held in this way can be a powerful force for integration. The financial aspect enables a fair energetic transaction. Here, money is not a means of manipulation, but rather it allows the empowered sex worker to have a balanced and satisfying life. In turn, these favorable conditions allow the workers to become vectors of healing for their clients. Integration thrives on win-win situations.

The Pivotal Piece of Empowerment

Chaitanya's story contrasts with Anne-Marie's story of disempowered sex work. When the container, the conditions, and the boundaries are not supported, sex work practiced from a disempowered place is clearly harmful to someone's body and psyche and reinforces the process of fragmentation. In Anne-Marie's case, the sexual experience is clearly not designed for either person to connect to their body or true essence. It is a damaging experience for everyone involved. Ultimately, the humanity of both parties gets eroded. Conversely, when practiced from a place of empowerment, sex is not only liberating and deeply healing for the person, but also allows empowered sex workers to create a healthier sexual context for all. With their knowledge, and in Chaitanya's case, her many years of kundalini yoga training and meditative practice, empowered sex workers become important healing catalysts and teachers, creating a better future for sex and connection in the world.

Soul Reverb

Now that you've experienced the worlds of empowered and disempowered sex workers, it's time for reflection. Get your journal or workbook out and jot down your answers.

1. Do you feel any kinship to Anne-Marie's or Chaitanya's story? In what ways do they remind you of your life?
2. What was most surprising for you in these two stories? What did you experience in contrasting these two stories?
3. Describe your relationship to sex, money, and healthy boundaries.

Chapter Affirmations:

- It is safe to honor my body, have boundaries, and have all my needs and wants met simultaneously.
- I celebrate the power of my sexual expression, for it is healing. I am empowered to create my own safe container for sexual healing.
- When I give myself permission, it gives permission to others.

Sex Up Your Life

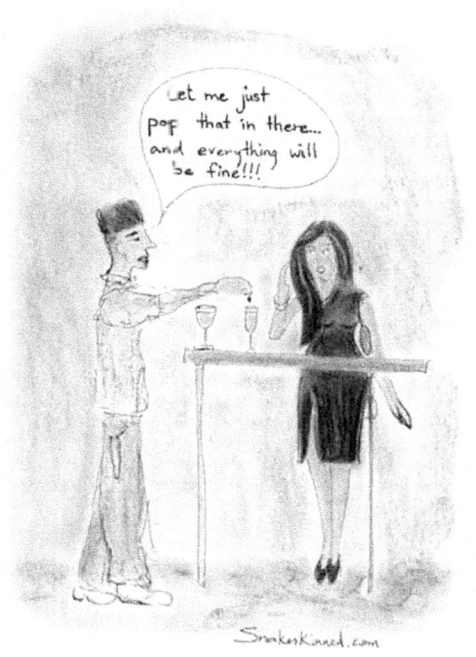

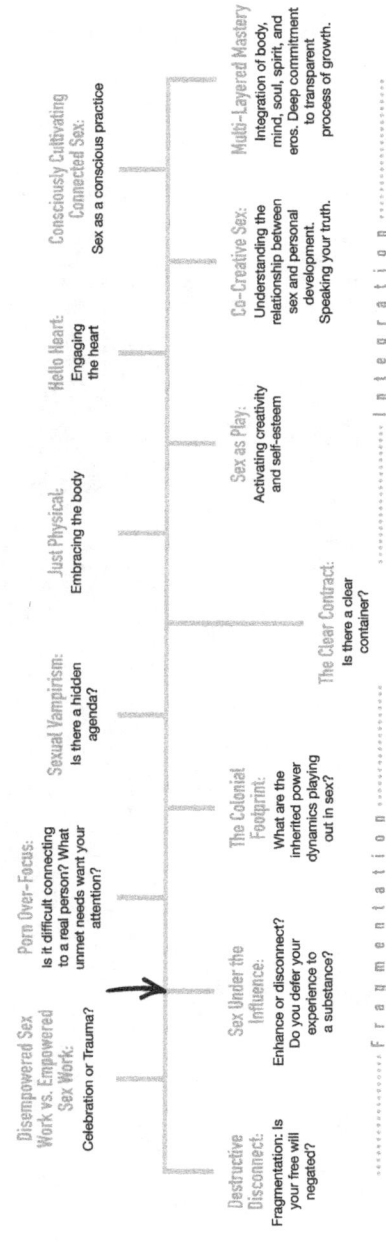

CHAPTER 3:

SEX UNDER THE INFLUENCE

"That's the problem with drinking, I thought, as I poured myself a drink. If something bad happens, you drink in an attempt to forget; if something good happens, you drink in order to celebrate; and if nothing happens, you drink to make something happen."

—Charles Bukowski

Now that we've explored what it looks like to engage in disempowered and empowered sex work, and qualities that differentiate the two, let's consider what happens with sex under the influence.

What does sex under the influence even mean, and how do you know you're engaging in it? We've all been to places where there were plenty of opportunities to indulge the senses. At what point does it become problematic?

Let's dive in!

In this chapter you will:

1. Learn what sex under the influence means
2. Experience Samantha's story of sex under the influence
3. Explore the dynamics involved with substances
4. Identify what it means to defer your power in this context

What is Sex Under the Influence?

Have you ever woken up beside someone—the name completely escapes you—and in a panic, try to unscramble your brain for any recall of last night? The litany of questions spews from your foggy mind. How did we/you get here? You may be surprised to find yourself naked beside this person. Maybe you wake up and the person is gone, but you can't for the life of you remember when they left! And did you have sex with them: yes or no?? You can't recall if you enjoyed it or if the other person enjoyed it! And when you sober up, you might start wondering if you are actually happy about what happened.

Sex under the influence involves being on a state-altering substance during sex. At its most base denominator, it includes the "get-drunk, get-laid" mentality. A lot of people turn to alcohol and recreational drugs to relax and entertain themselves, and maybe let their hair down to have fun, which obviously can work. Some swear by the libido-activating properties of their cherished substances. If you utilize recreational drugs or alcohol in a sustainable way, this may work for you.

Where it can become a little tricky is that as it loosens your inhibitions, it can also start impacting discernment, your connection to self and awareness of what is happening to you. If indulged in beyond your personal threshold, it can also make you black out and forget what happened—the good, the bad and the ugly. When under the influence, you are not fully connected to yourself, which makes it more challenging to connect with someone else. As we explore sex on this Continuum of Connection, the question boils down to this: when does the substance enhance your connection to your partner and when does it reduce it? And at what point do you give up your power to the substance itself?

Let's get acquainted with Samantha's story of sex under the influence and use that as a starting point for the discussion.

A heads up: There are some graphic descriptions in this story that may be disturbing to some.

Samantha's Story - On Taking Back Power

Samantha is a beautiful model with sex appeal oozing out of her golden skin, and yet, as far as she could remember, sex had been a very difficult and uncomfortable journey for her. I became fascinated with her story since it seemed to contradict the idea that sex must be an easy affair if you are beautiful and desired. As she shared her story with me, it became clear that in fact it had been quite the opposite: sex had been a trying experience in her life.

Her first sexual experience came in the form of an ultimatum. A boyfriend she met on her competitive swim team had sent her a letter saying, "I think I love you, but I'm not sure what love is." She described him as a "closed-off guy" with a really beautiful athletic body. He went on to write that he was ready for sex, and if she wasn't ready for it, they should break up. Samantha recalls feeling quite shut down from her own sexuality since the get-go. Being raised a Catholic in a prairie town meant she was supposed to save herself until she was married. Samantha recalls being reprimanded as a child for touching herself.

The message she got was that pleasure and genitalia must be quite the shameful combo. This discomfort combined with her boyfriend's ultimatum triggered some anxiety, and she thought, *if I don't comply, he will leave me.*

This dynamic also caused some of her fears around abandonment to flare up, feelings that had been ingrained from birth. Samantha describes being rejected from her mother's womb three months early as a premature baby and left to the sterile environment of an incubator; deprived of human touch. Her little self had already received a powerful message: my needs will not be met! This message was then consolidated through various family dynamics. For one, when her parents divorced, her mother was quite angry that Samantha had opted to live with her alcoholic father rather than her. On the day Samantha was packing up, her mother took all her luggage and threw it on the driveway as a symbolic statement, saying, "Fine, good luck!" To Samantha, it meant that she couldn't count on her mother anymore.

As for sex, Samantha recalls that for most of her twenties, she never felt like she really had a choice: "I didn't know how to make sex a mutual agreement." Being a very sensitive girl growing up amidst a lot of insecurity, "people pleasing" became her strategy to feel emotionally and physically safe. If she went along with what people wanted of her, everything would be okay. But as it turned out, people-pleasing would be costly throughout her life.

Samantha's first experience with sex happened one weekend where she had been drinking beer with her perfectly chiseled swim-team boyfriend at his parent's cabin. It was one of those awkward moments where neither of them knew what they were doing and where she felt like sex was just "happening" to her. She recalls not feeling totally happy with the situation. And because this first sexual experience happened within the confines of an ultimatum, it tainted how she felt. She didn't feel totally free or safe. Furthermore, drinking alcohol before having sex had also left a certain impression on her, one of awkwardness, a disjointed sexual exchange, and Samantha doesn't recall pleasure being part of the equation. This unsettling experience was her introduction to sex.

Family turmoil and financial stress put pressure on her swimming practice and she burned out. She missed the Olympic cut. This coincided with Samantha's discovery of the festive, underground world of raves, which had a definite appeal and intrigue for her. She could dress up with baggy pants, knot her hair into multiple buns, wear furry tops and glossy makeup and commune with a new family of wild revellers; a stark contrast to her disciplined life at the pool. She recalls feeling a sense of belonging there, a surrogate for the void left by her disintegrating family and the rash behavior of her alcoholic father. Her peers all came from dysfunctional families—all rejected from their families. Everyone was somewhat broken, hurting inside, and from this came a sense of camaraderie and solidarity. It was also a scene where taking drugs was a binding agent for the community. "We would always end up at the rave doing drugs together," she says.

Furthermore, she had dyed her hair blonde and, moving away from her demanding fitness training, her body softened. A stunning feminine form appeared, attracting the envy, jealousy and desires of many, which also spelled out many problematic dynam-ics to come. Her next sexual experience would happen within the rave context involving GHB, a date-rape drug.

It was just another rave weekend down at the bingo hall and Samantha had been hanging out with a group of guys, which included Michael, the guy who bragged about getting new timers onto cocaine and other substances. He offered Samantha a line to sniff. "I don't know," she said. "It is a rule I have for myself. I don't put things up my nose." "Why?" Michael asked. "Everyone else is doing it!" The guys were looking at her; they were all high, including one of them she was really attracted to. "Just try a little bit; if you don't like it, then you'll know." He upped the pressure. "Come on, you'll be fine; we're having fun!" She thought about it and gave in.

After taking a tiny line of it, her thoughts instantly started racing. She had an urge to change her clothes and went to her room where she tried on five different outfits: permutations of dresses and coats. She tried on everything she owned that could be worn at a rave. She started feeling anxious, even a little paranoid. Nothing happened that night.

But Michael sought her out another weekend. This time he offered Samantha a capful of GHB in liquid form. He told her it was the size ravers commonly did. They were going to have some fun. What she didn't know was that GHB was stronger in liquid form. Then, their common friend Patrice left the room, which left her alone with Michael in a vulnerable state. She started to feel dizzy and sweaty. She ran to the bathroom and started vomiting, plugging up the sink in Michael's bathroom. She tried cleaning it up but couldn't get rid of it. She remembered how nice Michael was about it, though. "Don't worry about it," he said and led her back to the room and pressed her body against a weight bench that was set up vertically.

He started kissing her clothes. The drug simulated a sexual feeling in spite of any true interest for sex at that moment; she was actually much too high to even function. She was conscious about what was happening, yet she had no access to her motor skills. She could barely hold herself up. Regardless, he started kissing her neck. She couldn't even talk and was unresponsive. He took off her pants and inserted his penis into her. She realized: "He was taking sex from me."

It wasn't consensual, and yet the memory of it was so foggy from being high. It was confusing and made her doubt her own perceptions. Had she given him the impression that it was okay? She had this way of giving others the benefit of the doubt, not trusting her own experiences and believing that other people always had her best interest in mind. In fact, a few months later when he asked to date her, she accepted. The notion of rape had not yet become a possibility in her own mind. This is not an uncommon experience for survivors of sexual assault: they doubt their experience and question whether they have the right to be upset.

The relationship went downhill from there. For six months, both heavily on drugs, Michael became mentally abusive to her, and she worried about her physical safety. She could see he wasn't well; he was smoking a lot of crack cocaine, had paranoia due to the selling of illegal drugs, plus he had been cheating on her. Samantha finally called it quits. He thought everyone was "stupid," and whenever she would speak up for herself by saying things like, "Well, I thought…," he would blast back at her with, "Yes, that is the problem, 'you' thought." But the break-up didn't go over well.

One day he arrived at her father's house where she had been staying, pounding on the door and trying to look into the windows, shouting, "I know you are in there, Samantha!" Her heart started racing. Thankfully she had a friend over, but they were both equally scared out of their wits. Michael had kicked through the screen door and was kicking the deadbolt door. The answering machine was filling up with messages on how she was a "fucking slut and a fucking whore" and how he was going to break her arms and legs. She knew she was neither of these insults. The next day they went to the police and a restraining order was put into effect. This concluded her relationship to Michael, but not this repeating storyline. This would repeat itself a few more times over the course of her life.

Fast forward to a few years later when, after entering the international modeling circuit, she found herself in Toronto where she met Daniel, a well-known "modelizer." He was this wealthy trust-fund kid who had no real job other than surrounding himself with models and other beautiful women, orchestrating a constant stream of partying for himself and his entourage and spending his money outrageously to bolster his social currency.

He knew every bar and club owner in the city and would reserve sectioned-off VIP tables raised on platforms to reinforce his socialite standing. Whoever was at his table was dressed to kill, and Samantha remembers how everyone would look at them: "You felt fabulous, living the luxurious and elaborate lifestyle of champagne and cocaine." Samantha had never had access to this type of abundance and prestige and concedes that at the beginning it was really exciting. Daniel loved taking photos beside all his fabulous friends and documenting his extravagant bacchanalian nights. He was always driving around town in white limos with beautiful women and rich men.

He was awkwardly intelligent, would get people on his level fast, pick them apart after only a couple of hours, and use it to manipulate them. "He could fuck with people," she said. "He knew who was weak and who wasn't. It thrilled him to be the puppet-master." No one had anything good to say about him, and yet he had a prosperous entourage. Samantha remembers that he was high most of the time with weed, but loved doing cocaine as well; it would make him crazy.

One night partying in his private home, while everyone else was consuming drugs in the basement common room, he had been caught pulling an unconscious woman's body by the arms up the stairs towards a bedroom. The man who saw him told him that if he caught him doing that again, he'd make sure he couldn't get back into the bars. Regardless, Daniel was not held accountable for his actions. Although whispers were starting to circulate about Daniel's behavior, no one had the courage to actually take a stand. The #MeToo movement was born out of calling out such behaviors to create a context where this is no longer tolerated. In retrospect, Samantha sees how, in spite of this incident, Daniel had started grooming her as a future target.

He decided to invite Samantha to join him as his assistant at Art Basel in Miami, one of the major artistic happenings in the world. This sounded really exciting to Samantha. "This is so cool," she thought. "I go for free. I get access to great art and the trip is complimentary!" With a father always concerned with money in their humble prairie existence, this elite jet-set world was mesmerizing and intoxicating to her. She decided to join him. But as soon as she got into the taxi in Miami, the vibe changed. When they had been packing, she locked the cat in the bathroom by accident.

When Daniel got in the taxi, he said: "I don't remember seeing kitty anywhere…" He then called his friend back in Toronto to check around and turned to Samantha and said, "You are one fucking idiot." This felt really violent to her. It reminded her of how her father could switch on a dime. She wanted to get out of the car and just leave. This had been a bad idea from the start. But then he apologized, and she found herself being swayed back into compliance by his words. Regardless, the whole weekend made her feel like she was a prisoner in a fancy jail. "He dragged me around to every art installation on the beach; whatever he wanted to do, I had to do it with him." When someone is being groomed, it is not uncommon to feel imprisoned and afraid to question anything.

One night, she had been walking all day with a new pair of boots that he had bought for her and her feet were hurting. She decided to leave the club early and head back to their hotel. "He called me and lost it on me." He told her he had paid for the trip, and she wasn't allowed to go home. No matter how much she was in pain, she had to stay with him. She hung up the phone, upset.

The next day, out of nowhere, she woke up laying beside him, and both were naked. She couldn't remember how she had gotten there. "Daniel said the night before I had grabbed these condoms and was like begging him for sex." But Samantha knew herself: she never begged anyone for sex. It didn't add up, but she couldn't remember anything. "I had a really bad feeling in my stomach. It didn't make sense." She never had been attracted to him and had pushed away his aggressive advances in the past. She couldn't figure out if she had been drugged, and she had no proof that he had in fact taken advantage of her. Once she got back to Toronto, she felt broken. She was confused with shame and decided to head back to her prairie town.

By the time I interviewed Samantha, she had done a lot of inner work on herself. She was well aware that she had grown up in a toxic family that had eroded her sense of healthy boundaries. Her alcoholic father could be quite manipulative and made her feel responsible for all the wrongs in his life, and she knew that some part of her had taken it on as her own responsibility. This meant that whenever someone accused her of something, she would doubt her own experience, and part of her would think it was indeed her fault, making her susceptible to being a victim of sexual assault.

She had never experienced "safe belonging" growing up. If there was any hint of losing her connections, Samantha would cave into other people's agendas, wanting to believe they had her best interest in mind when in fact they were blatantly taking advantage of her. She also had to look into the roots of her own addictive behaviors, which clearly had some anchoring in growing up with an alcoholic father. She became aware that she had followed some of his footsteps in how she dealt with her own life.

Learning to trust herself was a hard lesson that she would have to revisit a few times in her life. In fact, her healing journey involved the very process of taking back the power she had deferred to boyfriends, to other people's projections onto her and to drugs and partying. It meant finding the seat of her power, trusting herself and knowing how to hold solid boundaries.

But most of all, she had to relearn to value her inherent worth, regardless of external validation. Her journey of self-love was the cornerstone to revamp her life to a whole new level of satisfaction and connectedness to self. She did this through various self-development programs, healing work, coaching, Akashic Records work, yoga training, and female empowerment workshops on a wide variety of subjects including reclaiming women's pleasure. This deep work led her to the wholesome and loving partner she has today.

An important element to her process was weeding out the social scene that was fueled by drugs and alcohol. She knew she had to get these habits out of her life, that she didn't do well with drugs, and accept that losing most of her "party" friends would be part of the process.

This was necessary if she was serious about bringing her life to another level of authenticity, health and satisfaction. She managed to overcome these harsh realities while finding strength in her softness and wisdom.

Sex, Drugs, and Alcohol

In Samantha's story, we can recognize that drugs and alcohol have a confusing and numbing effect, whereby she and the entourage lose sense of themselves. With drugs and alcohol, sense perceptions get distorted. The self becomes less aware of one's own personal sense of agency and boundaries. It blurs reality, disconnects them, can even knock them out. In this context, presence to pleasure becomes tenuous, or simply impossible to experience. When someone is wasted, meaning they aren't totally "there," their consciousness and embodiment have been diminished. You can legitimately wonder, "Who is actually having sex?

When You Exit

For some, drugs and alcohol completely numb them from their feelings and bodily experiences. These substances are a quick exit out of their body, meaning consciousness leaves the body. Strangely, doesn't this sound like the previous chapters? "You leave your body." With assault, you leave your body unconsciously as a survival mechanism to survive cruelty. Here, taking a substance can be a means to check out as well. The only difference is that you are the one making the choice to take the substance. Of course, as seen before, you can also be coerced, groomed or deceived into taking drugs or alcohol. You may have witnessed this yourself: someone using drugs or alcohol to get into someone's pants. In these types of scenarios, we can see how substances are used intentionally to weaken another person's faculties and exercise of free will.

When No One Is Home

As seen in the story, if you aren't fully there, it also means you lose your capacity to make lucid choices and establish proper boundaries. When no one is home, it is hard to make a conscious decision, right? It's hard to decide who comes in and who doesn't. If there is no ego at home, who is there to ensure respect in the household?

Where is this invisible line between having fun and checking yourself out? If you are checked out, chances are you are not sufficiently present to experience much connection nor pleasure. For a mindful and connective experience to happen, you do need to be "home" rather than "out."

On Disconnection

As for the actual experience of connection and quality of sex, it has been documented that as the alcohol levels rise in the bloodstream, alertness, reaction time, and fine motor skills decrease, while clumsiness and slurred speech increase. Since good connective sex involves fine motor skills, the quality of the execution will obviously be affected. It also means that one's awareness and responsiveness to the other person's needs decline, which diminishes joint connectivity and interaction. This dynamic can find its parallel with other types of drug use. By de facto, one can say that sex under the influence, past a certain threshold, isn't designed for connection.

Substances to Enhance

Drugs and alcohol don't always end in such unfortunate and extreme stories. Some people skillfully use substances to enhance their reality rather than distort it, and there is a long history of people seeking out substances for aphrodisiacal properties. In David Deida's book[9], he talks about a woman whose consumption of alcohol actually allowed her to open up and experience a higher state of sexual pleasure.

Some acquaintances of mine swear by the powerful orgasm they access when taking drops of cannabis oil with chocolate and have playfully launched a line of "sexy chocolates" for middle-aged couples looking to re-ignite their sex life. Some people, with a strong grounding in mindful practice, even manage to use various psychoactive substances intentionally (or with ritual/ceremony) to access deeper sexual and spiritual experiences. Achieving this involves a lot of presence and relies on a conscious and awake practice for this to be successful, also proper dosing and pharmacology!

When the Captain Leaves the Ship

To propel sex into the upper spectrum, meaning for it to become a positive, integrative force in your life, sex requires consciousness and free will. As detailed in Chapter 1, consent is the very expression of your free will. However, consent can only be given if you are present enough to give it. As your intoxication levels increase,

---

9 Deida, David. (1995) Intimate Communion. Health Communication Inc.

your capacity to consent diminishes proportionately. If you've checked out and your consciousness dims, your free will no longer has dominion over your body.

This means the captain has left the ship. But even if you've left your ship, luckily from the standpoint of the law, it doesn't mean that any old pirate can come and take it over. "Legally that means, as explained here to Carleton University students, that if the person you're with is wasted, they can't say yes to sex—even if they still possess the ability to speak without slurring their speech." The law recognizes that intoxication puts you in a vulnerable state and that you require protection.

On Deferring Your Power

Nevertheless, we can all agree that if you are "not there," regardless of the legal safeguards, it still opens the door to unconscious and unfortunate things to happen to you. Your "I" is not there to be the gatekeeper of what you want and don't want. Psychoactive substances dim your consciousness and awareness. Your "I" may be on a nice trip, without bringing your body along! And to exercise your free will, your body and your "I" need to be working together. You need to know what is going on. Here, you lose access to your free will, even if you willfully took the substances. Now, that is something to get your mind around. What does this mean? It means that you are deferring your power to the substance. The substance is now guiding the experience in lieu of you.

On Sovereignty

If people want to mindfully use substances in support of deeper connection to self and others, it needs to be embedded in a conscious and solid practice to stay rooted in reality. It also requires them to be honest with themselves. Do they feel more embodied in themselves? Are the effects lasting? Do they ride waves, then crash? Does it help them build a stronger connection to self or others?

They need to evaluate whether it is giving them the skills to connect at that higher plane, or if it is simply becoming a crutch to avoid the "work," so to speak. When someone has found a substance that does turn them on, that enhances their experience and allows them to enjoy sex, in order to maintain their sovereignty, they also need to explore why this is not happening for them without the substance.

The Challenge

Find the natural path to these satiating and exciting sexual experiences to avoid becoming dependant on the substances in order to have them. Over the course of time, doses need to increase to mitigate the dulling effects of drug tolerance. Ultimately, being dependent on a substance for your sexual pleasure steals you of your connection to self and your inner investigation to find out how to get there, without any altering substances.

Our sexual energy is designed to flow: it's essentially life force that needs to move through our bodies. Blocking that energy has consequences. I will be exploring that theme in more depth in the Upper Continuum. It is a symptom of something greater that is calling our attention. It is telling us something about ourselves, about our partner, about our relationship, and it wants to be heard. It wants to be understood. If you jumpstart your sexual drive, appetite and pleasure with psychoactive substances, you may be avoiding the deeper work being called for here.

Psychoactives have been successfully used in various therapies when a trusted and trained practitioner guides the participants on a healing journey. Here, there is a trained practitioner that you trust guiding the healing journey. It also means that once you have "healed", you no longer need to use the substance once the issue has been addressed. It is a means for recovery.

My ultimate commitment is to inner freedom. True "sexual" sovereignty requires that you learn how to move your sexual energy yourself, unassisted. By taking this challenge, you will learn a lot about yourself. You will learn what's in the way and what needs to be addressed. You will learn about transformation, honesty, vulnerability. This is the initiation of passing the thread through the eye of the needle and will be dealt with in more depth in Chapters 10, 11, and 12, with Co-Creative Sex, Conscious Cultivation, and the Path of Mastery.

Human Freedom

Regardless, we come back to the concept of personal freedom. We are all free to choose our own path. It doesn't have to be a straight line, especially when we want to explore things for ourselves. And who knows what knowledge you will collect in having experiences. Embodied knowledge involves testing our limits, taking risks, and having novel experiences that we are drawn to. From there, we can make our own conclusions.

Nonetheless, our best ally is lucidity. When you are stuck in illusions, at some point, they will catch up to you. Eventually, the cracks reveal themselves. If you delude yourself in believing that someone is your friend, when they are not, eventually you will find out, and awakening to this will likely be painful. Sometimes a substance can appear to be a friend, and it may be just that in that moment, when later it may appear as an obstacle to overcome, something to leave behind to move along.

To Sum It Up

You may take state altering substances to help you out, but there's no guarantee. It's a gamble. On one hand, it could be a magical, hypnotic, soothing experience—perhaps just what you needed. In some cases, it may even be medicine for you. On the other, it could be hell on earth with blurry vision, chills, extreme paranoia, anxiety or worse. Just like rolling the dice, the substance decides what to do with your state of being: some are predictable uppers or downers, while the effects can also differ from person to person. You may wake up blissfully content, or you could be the victim of energy theft or even rape. Here, your free will has essentially been submitted to the substance.

Which leads us to the real issue: deferring your power to the substance. Power, or your agency, comes from fully taking responsibility for yourself, on all levels of your being. This means body, mind, soul, spirit, and sex. Power comes from engaging all your inner resources to experience those higher states. And this is, ultimately, an inner job. The more you re-integrate the parts of your being previously fragmented, the more inner power you access, the more you experience your full integrity. Meaning, your body needs to feel safe to be embodied, you need to trust your gut to make decisions, to create you must access your power, to feel you must open your heart, and to speak your truth your voice needs to resound. If you give up your power to a substance, you don't know where that substance is going to bring you, or you may not know how to integrate what you experienced into your conscious life. When you are no longer the ship's captain, something else takes over, whether pirate or tempest, and who knows what will happen to your ship!

Soul Reverb

Now that you're seeing Sex Under the Influence, it's time for reflection. Reach for your workbook or journal and write down your answers.

Take a Moment and Notice:

1. Where do you defer your power in your life? Is it to friends/family/colleagues, to romantic/sexual partners, to alcohol or drugs?
2. What does it look like? What beliefs do you have that lead you to defer your power?
3. What are you hoping to achieve when taking substances? How do the substances help you? In what ways do they harm you? Do you see any trends?
4. Try to find the root cause: what needs are you trying to meet when doing this? What issues are you avoiding addressing? Is this a strategy to "survive" something unpleasant?

Chapter Affirmations

- When I take ownership of all my power, I access higher forms of connection.
- The more I connect deeply to myself, the more I connect deeply with my sexual partner.
- Loving myself truly means acknowledging and tending to my deepest needs.

SEX ON THE CONTINUUM OF CONNECTION

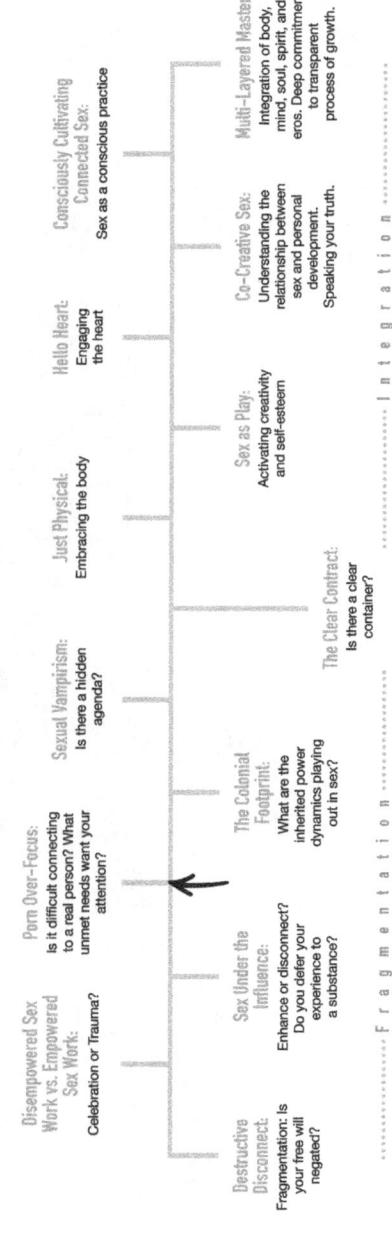

Disempowered Sex Work vs. Empowered Sex Work: Celebration or Trauma?

Porn Over-Focus: Is it difficult connecting to a real person? What unmet needs want your attention?

Sexual Vampirism: Is there a hidden agenda?

Just Physical: Embracing the body

Hello Heart: Engaging the heart

Consciously Cultivating Connected Sex: Sex as a conscious practice

Destructive Disconnect: Fragmentation: Is your free will negated?

Sex Under the Influence: Enhance or disconnect? Do you defer your experience to a substance?

The Colonial Footprint: What are the inherited power dynamics playing out in sex?

The Clear Contract: Is there a clear container?

Sex as Play: Activating creativity and self-esteem

Co-Creative Sex: Understanding the relationship between sex and personal development. Speaking your truth.

Multi-Layered Mastery: Integration of body, mind, soul, spirit, and eros. Deep commitment to transparent process of growth.

··········· Fragmentation ···········   ··········· Integration ···········

CHAPTER 4:

PORN-LITERATE MEETS PERSONAL DEVELOPMENT

"My reaction to porno films is as follows: After the first ten minutes, I want to go home and screw. After the first twenty minutes, I never want to screw again as long as I live."

—Erica Jong

So what about porn? How does it fall on this spectrum of connection? Like in all these various dynamics, porn is not a monolithic experience! With the advent of the internet, porn has stretched out in both directions: on one hand, you can find more and more degrading and extreme porn, but you can also find porn that is more connective and becoming increasingly interested in realistic portrayals of sex and female pleasure. It has also become interactive: made real-time with the advent of video-cams that anyone can clip onto their computer.

Here, you have the whole spectrum again. You have your powerful independent entrepreneurs behind their pixelated-screen making a killing with their unique versions of "effeuillage," often peppered with humorous banter and "friendly conversations". If we scoot down to the disempowered side of the Continuum, it can also be a portal into the lives of desperate poverty-stricken individuals from the four corners of the globe. In some cases, disenfranchised individuals in questionable conditions are broadcasting their genitalia for days on end to foreign audiences, with apparently scant financial returns.

As for the viewers: young and old alike, some are losing significant amounts of their sentient lives down this online portal, eclipsing any impetus for intimacy outside the blue-light of their devices. Others are simply curious or bored lurkers, looking for a momentous sexual excitement to pull them through a rough spot or amuse an idle moment. Some viewers express that their frequent visits have allowed them to even develop a form of intimacy with their preferred "Cam Girl". Considering these various circumstances, porn and camming—which involves live-streaming an erotic performance with a webcam—can play many different roles in people's lives. Depending on the actual dynamics, this can operate both as a fragmenting or integrating experience for those involved.

As we look deeper into the question of porn under its many guises, it is helpful to look at extremes to gain perspective. How about we look at porn when its starts overshadowing the intimacy in someone's life and starts resembling addiction? What does this dynamic reveal to us about porn, sex, and our capacity for relationships? And how about the consequences it has on people's lives? What are they trying to achieve with their acute consumption of porn? It begs the question, "What needs are wanting to be met?" So let's dive in and see what porn has to teach us about connection and disconnection.

A heads up: There are some graphic descriptions in this chapter that may be disturbing to some.

Sex Up Your Life

In this chapter you will:

- Explore what it means to be "porn-literate"
- Learn the light and shadow sides of the porn industry
- Experience Mark's story of struggle with porn
- Learn how porn can positively and negatively affect your relationship
- Identify some of the core symptoms of porn over-focus and its consequences

How people choose to express their sexuality is a huge emotional trigger for many. Porn is one of those subjects that elicits a visceral response. It may be frowned upon perhaps because of the discomfort it may awaken in someone or it is adamantly and aggressively defended because someone dared flirting with the mere idea of criticizing it. It is a touchy subject.

According to the Merriam-Webster dictionary, pornography is defined as "the depiction of erotic behavior—in printed or visual materials—intended to cause sexual arousal". In itself, this is not a problem. Erotic art has been documented throughout history, found on the walls of Egyptian pyramids, sculpted into onyx in ancient Rome, formed into terra cotta plates in Mesopotamia. And what about the millennial old sexy Khajuraho temples with their array of juicy erotic positions sculpted into stone from ancient India? Sexual arousal is part of the human experience. Erotic ideas and fantasies beg to be imagined! The difference between erotic art and porn is that porn is designed to trigger a powerful chemical response in your brain, which requires more examination to better understand the full impact on our lives.

A 2017 PornHub year-in-review report suggests that "every five minutes, PornHub transmits more data than the entire contents of the New York Public Library's 50 million books." This kind of consumption would be the envy of any major library of the world. Obviously, these video files are a highly sought-after media by many. According to PornHub, the demographic breakdown is 75 male users to 25 percent female.

So why does porn have such appeal and why does it have the capacity to trigger such intense criticism and aggressive retaliations?

If you consider that Abraham Maslow's self-actualization pyramid lists sex as a basic need[10], the dots start to connect. Any threat to a basic need will necessarily trigger a survival mechanism.

When someone has an acute or loaded response to something, it basically speaks to the fact that somewhere in the recesses of their being, whether it be conscious or unconscious, something is flaring up. Today, for people working in the field of sexuality, there is a wide-spanning consensus that most people in the world need some form of healing around sexuality. If the state of sex were all fine and dandy, sex wouldn't be such a taboo subject. We wouldn't be seeing all kinds of misaligned expressions of sexuality overpopulating our media and court systems! We'd also have a holistic, effective, and inspiring sex education to introduce such a powerful phenomenon for those coming of age. For the most part we don't.

When sexual impulses and expression have been thwarted or shamed, a malaise will show up as a survival tactic. It will show up in how we react emotionally to it as well. This is why some people will rail angrily against anyone trying to get in the way of their strategy to appease their needs as they play out in sexuality. This is the strategy they have elected to foster "comfort" and "satisfaction" for themselves, i.e. how they "soothe" themselves. They will want to protect it at all costs.

On the other hand, if someone shuts porn out with the same level of vehemence, it also expresses something. This is because sexuality also touches on questions of emotional safety: safety to

---

10 "Maslow's Hierarchy of Needs". simply psychology. Retrieved 8 November 2018.

be respected and be treated well. If someone watches porn that seems dehumanizing to them, they may be worried of being dehumanized themself during sex. It may trigger antipathy for porn, and by extension, for sex.

Basically, how we react to something reveals our worries, fears, and injuries. Acknowledging these subtler dynamics helps us have a more constructive conversation about porn.

Porn: Healthy or Unhealthy for Sexuality?

On the subject of connectivity, I find it best to contextualize porn to understand the personal responses we have and their deeper meaning. Some people seek porn as a way of educating themselves, looking for creative ideas, inspiration, or perhaps permission to explore. Some simply want to get sexual with their partner, and porn does the trick! For many tweens, porn is a window into what sex looks like, as they try to wrap their mind around sex.

Others utilize porn because they are looking to meet some of their unmet basic needs, at times "urgent", which is the fulcrum point where we tip into the realm of the hungry ghost, a term used in Buddhism to characterize individuals driven by intense emotional needs. Some turn to porn because it gives them a release of tension, a peak of pleasure. It gives them that much sought after energy "hit" when they are otherwise feeling depleted. Some watch porn to relax as they would take a glass of wine or a beer on a Friday night. Others will watch it to get hammered and forget their week altogether!

The good news about pornography is that porn interested in female pleasure has entered the market, and the work of Erika Lust is such an example. In fact, according to the 2017 Pornhub Year-in-Review, one of the three top searches has been "porn for women." The more contentious news, as described by Gail Dines in

Porn-literate Meets Personal Development

Pornland: How Porn Has Hijacked Our Sexuality, is an increasing amount of extremely offensive and denigrating porn being produced, including "rape porn," which may crank the imagination of unhealthy and unstable people, potentially putting others at risk as a result of viewing it. Or as Kate Julian put it in her article "Why Are Young People Having So Little Sex", it may be simply "scaring people off" from sex altogether due to some of the more sensitive sexual behaviors being replicated by un-experienced individuals, notably anal sex without lubrication, erotic asphyxiation without consent, or simply ejaculation on the partner's face without preparation. But the extreme content goes far beyond these forms of activities.

The Exodus Cry website has collected many horrific stories of women being "assaulted on camera for profit at the hands of Kink"—the iconic San Francisco BDSM porn studio that shut down in 2017. According to Exodus Cry, the studio's practices included "flogging, whipping, caning, electrocution, submersion in water, cutting, hog-tying, defecating on, urinating on, public humiliation, and simulations of gang rape to name a few."

To flip the script for a moment, according to an article in the Guardian, others lament the closing of such an iconic place. For them, Kink.com has worked to de-stigmatize BDSM. "It's heartbreaking," said Lorelei Lee, a longtime Kink performer. "To lose this in a city that is losing resources for artists and queers and sex workers in such a huge way is sad." The article explains that Kink.com "built its reputation as the rare porn company with a mission statement – to "demystify and celebrate alternative sexualities by providing the most ethical and authentic kinky adult entertainment."

Online traffic reveals this type of porn is still very much in demand, while Kink.com simply closed because of the new competitive realities of the online market, rather than its edgy practices. In the "Conscious Kink" chapter of this book, we will take a look at how BDSM can be used in very effective and integrative ways. But, one can also be weary of the downsides that may be incurred when footage of pain are unleashed into the online landscape without any guidance or concern. Results can be alarming.

I have been haunted by the idea that Bradley Barton, the truck driver arrested for the death of Cindy Gladue—a Métis woman found dead in a motel bathtub with an 11-centimetre-long lesion to her vaginal wall—had watched sites on how to insert very large objects into women's genitalia. Copy cats of violent sexual behaviors are real and can emulate damaging scenarios with devastating and troubling results.

In fact, with the advent of free streaming porn populating the internet, the income generating opportunities have restructured themselves around offering exclusive material, whether through exclusive live cam-shows, or through offering niche content capitalizing on these extreme portrayals of sex designed to push the envelope and pull in clients willing to pay for "added value".

Nonetheless, the important thing, as Caia Hagel, co-author of *Girl Positive*, puts it, is to become porn-literate. In her book, she makes a good case with her co-author, Tatiana Fraser, that the most empowering way of addressing porn and sexuality with young people is by fostering a safe space for conversation where their experiences are valued and recognized, which by extension is also true for adults. Who doesn't appreciate a safe space to speak their vulnerable truth?

This way you build your sexual identity from the inside out in a supportive environment rather than via shame, or unspoken expectations. Your voice counts. Your individuality is essential to the process and outcome. When chastising porn as "bad," we find ourselves bogged down by the shame game once more. Therefore, these collective and supportive conversations allow for one to grow into oneself in a safe way.

Part of the porn-literate conversation must address commercial interests in order to get a clearer picture of what economic forces are driving the industry. In 2001, the porn industry was grossing billions annually and, according to *Forbes* magazine, market share could be broken down like this: : adult videos ($1.8 billion), internet ($1 billion), magazines ($1 billion), pay-per-view ($128 million), and cell phones ($30 million). According to the Irish Examiner, in 2012 the industry was grossing a nice 14 billion. Estimates greatly fluctuate from one source to the next. Getting numbers for this industry is always a tricky endeavour, considering that there is often undisclosed income. These rough estimates show that the industry has the possibility of being quite lucrative.

Since 2012, the porn industry has considerably restructured itself with the flooding of the online market with pirated material and the creation of porn tubes streaming free materials. Many 'traditional" porn studios have actually shut down, and tech savvy entrepreneurs behind online hubs such as MindGeek have taken over the market with their free streaming platforms. This shift is comparable to the highjacking of TV with Netflix and radio via Spotify, which creates a monopoly where the studio must now go through these porn tubes to advertise their paid content for exposure. By acquiring the most popular websites from competitors, MindGeek now owns an estimated 8 out of 10 of the largest porn tubes, including PornHub, RedTube, and YouPorn.[11]

By redirecting the porn traffic to their tubes via free streaming material, this funnel-like economic model has become the clear winner of the industry: anyone wanting to rack in any profits must advertise on their "tubes" (so-called because of their similarity with YouTube). This includes porn studios and camming networks such as LiveJasmin and MyFreeCams if they want to garner any piece of the profit pie. According to the Luxembourg Times, in

---

11 Auerbach, David. (2014, Oct 23) Vampire Porn: MindGeek is a cautionary tale of consolidating production and distribution in a single, monopolistic owner, Slate. https://slate.com/technology/2014/10/mindgeek-porn-monopoly-its-dominance-is-a-cautionary-tale-for-other-industries.html

2015, MindGeek alone, reported 460 million dollars in revenue. With the restructuring of the market, some believe that the value of the porn industry now averages out at 5$ billion. Others believe that the market value has simply taken on a new face, especially when considering the advent of camming.

Douglas Richter, an executive-level consultant with LiveJasmin, one of the top cam sites—believes the annual revenue from camming to exceed $1 billion, making it the driving force of the adult industry. Although prerecorded movies and clips are still being produced, interactive entertainment, now account for a large part of all porn sales. The sites and the performers make their money through tips, resembling gambling coins that users buy. During this online peep show, the models receive tips to perform. They devise strategies, games, and coo-ing techniques to get the coins clinking, including reminding the men "just how sweet they are!", apparently one of the winning formulas. Tips can be as little as nil during a show, all the way up to record tips such as 260,000 tokens in one shot which means $13,000, as reported by "Mila, a 'somewhat blasé' German-born porn star working out of Thailand.

As the industry morphs, web-camming companies are another economic winner. Adjacent to a proliferation of personal ventures popping up from enterprising individuals, both men and women, are empowered to create their own pornographic material and cast themselves in the roles they design, and in the circumstances they chose. Some studios have jumped on the live-camming bandwagon as well, which means various types of "arrangements", dynamics, and struggles. In some less fortunate situations, this means variations on the themes of servitude and indentureship, depending on the levels of empowerment and economic freedom these individuals have at their disposal. The next technological revolution is on its' way with humanoid robots, high-performing sex dolls, and 3-D virtual technology expected to generate whole new streams of income generating opportunities for the porn industry, which, of course, means a whole slew of new engulfing virtual realities to experience and get lost in.

The Light and Dark Side of the Porn Industry

It is worthwhile taking a moment to think about the pornography industry, not only from an economic standpoint, but also within the context of the Continuum of Connection. Some actors love their job. Sexual expression is a celebration for many people. In the documentary film "Cam Girlz" (2015), women, including a vivacious older lady, express how much they enjoy sharing their sexuality online, how empowering it is for them, and how much fun they have. You can also get hints of the ups and downs one would experience with putting themselves out in such an intimate way, with the vagaries of inconsistent traffic, the emotional roller coaster that comes with the "likes" and "dislikes" of the social media age, and the trials of being self-motivated "solopreneurs". They also hint at the blurring of lines between the internet and real life meet-ups. Grey zones will necessarily appear, if we simply consider human nature! When people show up as empowered individuals celebrating their sexuality, and conduct themselves in a safe and respectful environment, with clearly set boundaries, the results appear to be a win-win scenario.

When boundaries get murky, and work conditions become exploitative, the negative side of the industry surface. Some of the harsher by-products for porn actors have been reported as STDs, drug abuse, various forms of exploitation, manipulation and pressure tactics and physically damaging film scenes (resulting in anal and uterine damage). There is also physical and verbal abuse, psychological trauma, physical exhaustion, dissociation due to the hardcore violence in some scenes, brainwashing, suicidality, and misleading actors into prostitution.[12, 13] In this type of disempowering environment, true connection clearly is not an objective on the film set, nor in the camming studio, and probably won't be for the viewers, regardless of their potential appeal. This is where the porn and camming industry become a machine of fragmentation, meaning a process that hurts us, numbs us, dissociates us, and where we lose access to parts of ourselves. It leaves us in shambles.

How the Shadow Side of Porn Affects Our Real Relationships

When watching porn that seeks to dehumanize, the consumer is often invited to identify with the alpha muscle male brandishing his large genitalia as he aggressively comes to a peak. In scenarios such as these, the viewers get a very skewed experience of what a mutually satisfying sexual experience looks like. It is a far cry from the plethora of techniques designed to pleasure women. Most men can orgasm in under five minutes, while experts tend to agree that women require on average twenty minutes. This is why it is generally prescribed to focus on a lot of foreplay for women to truly enjoy the sexual experience. Therefore, the porn scenarios are not always realistic portrayals of female pleasure, nor realistic portrayals of male appendages, which leaves many men thinking they are "short" of being truly effective or desirable when it comes to sex.

As for higher states of pleasure, according to Catherine Blacklege, author of *The Story of V: A Natural History of Female*

---

12 *10 Ex-Porn Performers Reveal the Brutal Truth Behind Their Most Popular Scenes (2019, May 22) Fight the New Drug.* https://fightthenewdrug.org/10-porn-stars-speak-openly-about-their-most-popular-scenes/

13 *Porn Star Elizabeth Rollings Escapes the Killer Porn Industry (2018, May 5) The National Center on Sexual Exploitation.* https://endsexualexploitation.org/articles/porn-star-elizabeth-rollings-escapes-the-killer-porn-industry/

Porn-literate Meets Personal Development

Sexuality, "studies show women need a mere one or two minutes, on average, to reach their second climax, also known as a multiple orgasm." In fact, "the most female orgasms observed was an impressive 134 in just 60 minutes." If someone decides to enact the pornified scripts where foreplay and the building of female arousal may have been omitted from the script, the results may not be as expected. The individuals may get a skewed idea of how to reproduce what is portrayed, and their expectations and fantasies may override a real person's experience, without considering if it is working for their sexual partner.

If we follow that a little deeper, this projection creates a wedge in the actual connection between the two partners. They are not truly connecting to their sexual partner but using their body as a prop to play out a part devised in their imagination. The sexual partner is likely to sense this disconnect. Furthermore, since they are not connecting to their partner, they can actually feel disappointed when the illusion ultimately fades away and their fantasies don't seem to play out as on the screen, falling short of the desired outcome.

In fact, there is growing evidence that some people are actually forgoing sex altogether, i.e. opting-out of sex with a human partner, because the "online libido" is way more satisfying, less complicated, and more "reliable" in its' pleasure inducing properties. In Kate Julian's article, she speaks of the "Herbivore Men", called the Soushoku Danshi in Japan, who are "ambivalent about pursuing either women or conventional success." She also cites Roland Kelts, a Japanese American writer and Tokyo resident, who has written about 'a generation that found the imperfect or just unexpected demands of real-world relationships with women less enticing than the lure of the virtual libido", which we can imagine is not a "made in Japan" only phenomena. The common theme that you find amongst people with sexual or relational trauma is fear of intimacy.

In researching about online addictions, I came across a case study of a 22 year-old Korean man with an isolating pathological gaming problem. His social skills remained undeveloped from a young age into adulthood. After therapy, he managed to come to grips with his gaming addiction that had literally taken over his life, but he hadn't succeeded in supplanting his excessive porn consumption with any real sexual rapport with another human being. When trying to deepen their understanding of what was happening, the researchers explained that they hit up against a wall, the topic being too touchy for him to talk about. Gaming and porn appear to have an interchangeable appeal, porn being "a-no-brainer" leap for the worldwide gaming subculture. In fact, PornHub reports a 60% increase in traffic when "Fortnite," a popular online game, shut down their site for a twenty-four hour emergency maintenance.

In cases where people opt-out of intercourse with another human being, they are trading in the effort required to establish any true intimacy with a person "in the flesh," for the controllable and safe fantasy of the virtual world. There is a lot less "skin" in the game if you are simply masturbating alone in a room with a screen. Usually, dealing with another person involves mutual growth, understanding, communication skills, and a need for introspection. A real person involves being confronted with oneself. In rubbing up against the discomfort of our edges with another, we discover how we must grow to achieve connection. This is the place where we need to dive into our vulnerabilities. When dealing uniquely with the "fantasy" we have selected and can control, in which we are essentially the only player, we are retreating from the experience of true intimacy and the need to surrender to its powerful learning curve. The online libido can easily be looped, while other parts of our being remain stunted, unchallenged to grow, and over time, become atrophied.

Porn Over-Focus

Which begs the question, what about porn addiction? Does it exist? And what is the mechanism? The American Psychiatric Association has not included Internet Porn Addiction in their Manual of Mental Disorders (DSM), the "Bible" for diagnostic categories in mental health. Instead it has been flagged as requiring further study to better evaluate its legitimacy, the debate being along the line of: We can prove that individuals get pathologically addicted to substances, yet can we prove that "behaviors" alone are addictive as well?

And yet in 2013, the APA moved "pathological gambling" from being simply defined as an impulse disorder to a new category called: "Addiction and Related Disorders." Nigel Turner, a research scientist at the Centre for Addiction and Mental Health and the Department of Public Health Sciences at the University of Toronto, believes that "it de-emphasizes the substance per se and focuses more on the experience of the person. It also works towards an understanding of factors that make some people more vulnerable not just to a specific drug, but to any addictive behavior."

The few scientific reviews to be found on Internet Porn Addiction, are largely neuroscience studies that support the application of the addiction model to addictive internet-related behaviors and find it difficult to justify the APA's explicit disavowal of other compulsive internet behaviors.[14] They refer to many studies that show that behavioral addictions undergo very similar processes involving the reward centers of the brain, targeted by addictive substance such as cocaine. Volkow and al. describe three stages of the addictive cycle: 1. Binge/Intoxication 2. Withdrawal/Negative Affect 3. Preoccupation/Anticipation.[15] In this cycle, we have a process of reinforcement to avoid withdrawal, which then results

---

14 https://www.ncbi.nlm.nih.gov/pubmed/24904393#

15 https://www.ncbi.nlm.nih.gov/pmc/articles/PMC2805560/

in a tolerance increase as one seeks higher thresholds of stimulus for satisfaction. Some of the negative by-products are social and occupational neglect.

In the New York Times Best Seller *The Brain That Changes Itself*, psychiatrist and psychoanalyst Norman Doidge summarizes the research on addiction and the reward system. He states that the continued release of dopamine into the reward system when an individual compulsively and chronically watches internet pornography stimulates neuroplastic changes that reinforces the experience and eventually forms brain maps for sexual excitement.

Porn is designed to ignite pleasure and activate sexual drive, and many use it to masturbate and climax. It would be hard to imagine that experiencing such high levels of pleasure in response to these images wouldn't then in turn activate the reward centers and eventually restructure them according to these super levels of stimulus, also known in the scientific world as "supranormal stimulus."

While many viewers of adult content don't notice any negative impacts on their lives or on their sexual partners, porn can become problematic for others. The Kinsey Institute survey found 9 percent of porn viewers said they had tried unsuccessfully to stop. Some men I have talked to notice some of the damaging impacts on their lives. They describe having trouble enjoying sex with real women because of their over-consumption, which ultimately results in states of arousal exclusively when watching porn. Some experience loss of interest and desire for their actual partner. They acknowledge that they rely too heavily on porn, yet also can't imagine stopping. The issue here is not the porn itself, but the person watching the porn and what's going on in their thoughts and feelings. The thought of stopping, according to one man I talked to, would be "just too difficult"; it would need to be a process of slowly weaning off it, not dissimilar to using a patch to stop smoking.

On the flip side, for some, the use of porn can be a positive experience and a nice addition to their relationships. It can help them get over humps or issues with sexual shame. It can get a couple successfully aroused. When people manage to use porn as a tool to help them in foreplay or otherwise, the experience can be a win-win situation. The problem occurs when porn starts taking over the whole of your sexual experience, when you become dependent on it for sexual release, if it disconnects you from your partner, or if it isolates you because contact with another person appears to be unattainable or undesired. If porn becomes a diversion from your problems, it will start causing harm to you and your relationships and eventually affect your mental health. This is when porn tips into a process of fragmentation rather than integration.

So, let's dive into Marc's story and see what challenges he meets with porn.

Marc's Story—Struggles with Porn

When I started interviewing Marc, he was already well aware of the impact of porn on his life. He was clear that somehow it was warping his sense of sexuality and his relationship to the female body.

"I knew my own personal status was suboptimal, that it was unhealthy in some way. Sex was like a slave driver, and my mind was constantly looking for sex or sexuality, looking for the dopamine. I also knew it was based on a fiction, that it was plastic coded, not realistic, better-than-real-life, and a waste of time." Marc knew how it was impacting his marriage. He was actively looking for solutions and was authentically motivated by the idea of being a good lover for his wife.

He had grown up in a family where parental screaming matches were a family fixture. With a father who was often absent due to a suspected double life, and a stay-at-home mother who was imploding under feelings of abandonment and lack of support,

Marc remembers often retreating to his room because of the intensity of the conflicts in the house

At nine years old, in the back of his father's closet, he discovered porn. He developed quite the ninja strategy, hovering against walls, and making leaps across doorways to get into his father's closet without being seen, to watch it. The first time he actually ejaculated came as a surprise! What was that? All he knew was that it excited him. In high school, he had gotten into *Debbie Does Dallas* with his friends. No one masturbated while watching it, but once he was alone, he did.

In college, the advent of the internet meant porn was now at his fingertips. He had an open-door policy with his dorm buddy, which meant he could always go to his buddy's room to watch porn. "Mostly vanilla," he recalls, "with some threesomes, some lesbian porn, but mostly just hard-core sex between a man and a woman in different positions."

Looking back at his life, Marc could see how he was programming his body to get aroused to such images. He recognized that porn made it more difficult to cultivate a natural sexuality with a real woman. "I wanted to have sex with a woman and make it look like porn. I wanted it to be a stimulant and get the dopamine dump." But he also recognized that in porn there is no relating and no relationship. "I felt like to get to that point where a woman wants me like that, for us to get to that primal place, it's like going through a maze. There is no video for that."

By the time he hit his late twenties and thirties, his porn consumption went underground. It wasn't something he discussed, except for maybe the odd crass joke. "I never told my wife that I used porn, not that I hid it from her. She knew I used it sometimes. But I took steps so she wouldn't find out."

He became aware that he indulged in porn as a form of escapism when he felt other needs not being met and not speaking up about them. When he made the bold decision to stop consuming

Porn-literate Meets Personal Development

porn, he included his wife in the process. To his surprise, she was not offended nor uncomfortable broaching the subject. Moving forward, whenever he felt the urge or craving for porn, he would tell her, and they would approach it as a couple. Frankly, in the past, he would essentially do it to "jerk off." "It's like trying to get off drugs. You get a high, then you crash. Emotionally, you feel shattered, unstable. I would tell her that."

Marc knew he needed to find another route if he wanted to go farther with his wife. Every time he had the urge to watch porn, he says, "It was a reminder to me that I can just talk to her." But it didn't mean sex was any easier. He deeply struggled with finding how to connect sexually with her in a mutually satisfying way.

Once, they had been traveling after a fun birthday weekend and found themselves in a "Love Motel" on a stopover in Manila, Philippines. As they were stretched out on the heart-shaped bed, Marc took the remote control and started flipping through the stations. Some Japanese porn caught his eye: "What's that?" he thought. The women on the screen had her face scrunched up. Her voice shrilled as if in excessive pain. Marc and his wife started talking about it.

In the process of talking and watching, David recalls his wife getting pretty horny. And yet, it was "like she was angry too." They started having sex. When they were finished, her anger had subsided, but she related back to him that it had not fulfilled her at all.

Marc started researching and reading about desire, sex, and connection. He found different websites such as *www.yourbrainonsex.com* and *www.reuniting.info* where he started exploring the principles of Karezza, a gentle, affectionate form of intercourse in which orgasm is not the goal, and ideally does not occur in either partner while making love in search of mutually satisfying sex.

They dabbled with open relationships in search of a better model. But ultimately, Marc felt like it took far too much effort navigating all the expectations involved for the disappointing returns. He also recognized that it was taking a toll on his energy levels. He was feeling drained. His true, deep desire was to find deep sexual connection with his wife. He wanted to be desired and appreciated by her, not by a whole slew of other people that were insignificant to him. He wanted to deepen the one relationship that was meaningful to him and that he had committed to. He wanted to feel like, in her eyes, he was the "hot shit" that she deeply craved and desired, and that he had the capacity to satisfy her.

As we wound down our interview process, Marc was still intensely searching to find that place of satisfaction with his wife. It wasn't proving to be a quick-fix solution and, in fact, was quite taxing and frustrating. This story is a good example of how our sexual energy is pushing us to grow, pushing us to dig a little deeper, understand something that seems beyond our grasp, beyond our current state of consciousness. Sexual energy has the power to uncover our truth if we let it. On our last call, Marc told me they had hired a marriage counsellor and that the work was arduous and ongoing. He didn't conceal that anger was now a surfacing reality for him.

Porn addiction, or porn over-focus, is actually a coverup for much deeper things going on. When we avoid seeing the truth of our pain or hurt, we start breeding non-realities to cope with our lives. In many cases, like Marc's, porn becomes a coping mechanism. Marc's strategy as a young boy had been to find comfort in a disquieting family dynamic. Yet eventually this strategy morphed into his dealing mechanism, and slowly into a habit, which, over time, distorted his relationship to sexual intimacy with the very person he wanted to have it with. In Marc's case, he started noticing his coping mechanisms and wanted to address them, but as it turned out, discovering this was only the tip of the iceberg. It was only the beginning of unraveling the other concealed issues.

So, what do we find under these non-realities? To name a few, we often find fear, rejection, anger, neediness, grief, abandonment, control, numbness, sorrow, pain, loneliness, and disconnection. Everyone has their own path to wholeness, and moves at their own speed, but it seems a more effective and efficient strategy to go to the root cause of the discomforts and try to heal it. Why waste precious time in non-realities? Why maintain a state of numbness if the problem can be solved by going deeper?

Symptoms of Porn Dependency

Regardless of whether it is an official mental health diagnosis, people experience feelings of dependency on porn consumption and struggle with various dynamics because of it. Pornography is comparable to an eating disorder. Food is not inherently bad, rather the issue is found in the individual's relationship to its consumption and whether or not this is a symptom of a deeper problem.

So, for the purpose of this book, I will address their complaints and feelings of dependency as a loss of sovereignty.

Psychologist and Professor Emeritus at Stanford University Philip Zimbardo talks about a "masculinity crisis" in his in-depth look into the lives of 20,000 young men and their relationships with video games and pornography. Young, isolated men are "combining playing video games, and as a break, watching on average two hours of pornography a week."

Dr. Zimbardo has documented young men expressing things like, "When I'm in class, I'll wish I was playing World of Warcraft. When I'm with a girl, I'll wish I was watching pornography, because I'll never get rejected." His data reveals that porn "begins to change brain function. It begins to change the reward center of the brain and produces a kind of excitement and addiction."

I personally feel this points to deeper questions. Why are these boys seeking porn at this scale? What needs are screaming to be met? If we consider that overconsumption of porn is used to fill in a void, of what then? If we consider that addiction is an attempt to bring well-being where there is lack of, what is causing this deficit? What is lacking in their lives? Is it poor self-esteem and social ease, underdeveloped capacity for connection and intimacy? Being truly seen and perceived? Not feeling adequate and enough to be loved by a real person?

Some men have shared with me that their over-consumption of porn has distorted their view of a woman's body, whether its having unrealistic expectations of what a woman's body should look like or because they have trouble seeing a woman's body without the pornified filter. They can no longer look at a woman's body as natural. Various body parts, most notably breasts, ass and crotch, become instant sexual triggers. Their eyes become magnetized to these places as they are drawn to get their hit. You can feel it when someone looks at you, or others, in this way. Suddenly, you are not an individual anymore but have become a body part that has triggered some fantasy. At times it can feel very uncomfortable and intrusive.

From an energetic standpoint, they have accessed your personal space without permission. This is why many women have started fighting for the right to reclaim their nudity without it being associated with anything sexual. Breasts are perfectly natural. "Free the nipple!" In many traditional societies, women were topless twenty-four-seven. Now, women need to assemble in protest, baring their breasts, to exclaim that "Nudity is Not Sexual." They are fighting to reclaim a safe space to experience their bodies outside of this pornified mindset.

Go Nude

On the flipside of this, feeling the sexiness of one's nudity is also a powerful experience, and many women love indulging in it! I've seen a proliferations of dance classes that invite women to express their sexiness, whether it be pole dancing, burlesque, or sexy events where they can dress up to enhance their nudity. And women are signing up in droves.

Women want to experience the sexiness of their curves, and the elixir of their sexual energy. If we consider this from the standpoint of integration, we need our sexual energy to be whole, because this is an important part of self-expression. This is true for both men and women.

At the end of the day, the question boils down to this: Is the dynamic that's playing out empowering? Is there mutual respect? Is it an authentic expression of yourself? If the answer is yes, all the more power to you! On the flipside, is there any manipulation, one-sidedness, or entitlement involved? Is your well-being esteemed? Are you deferring your value to someone else? To feel that true authentic power and inner value, you will most likely need to shed any limiting scripts found in the pornified mindset, notably reclaiming the script and the gaze and redefining it! Making it an "original" script that is simply an expression of you.

Of course, censorship is not the solution, as Michael Leahy, a recovering porn addict now on speaking tours, explains. "It isn't about censorship. I'm against censorship. I'm not interested in morality discussions, and I'm not here to tell anyone how to live their life. What I'm interested in is the facts about how pornography affects our brain chemistry, our physiology, and our relationships. I very much bought into that whole porn culture. I didn't think there was anything wrong with it, I didn't believe I was hurting anyone and yet eventually it would end up costing me a fifteen-year marriage, my two boys, and my career."

Again, in order to have a real conversation about porn, we must establish a safe space to have it. Once established, we can have a real conversation and talk about the real dynamics at play. Leahy's contribution to the discussion begs the following questions: Why can porn engulf us? Why do we turn to porn for satisfaction?

What needs are being expressed that need tending to? And how do we meet these needs most effectively?

Yet going deeper, for some people, can be a very scary process. *You mean I have to deal with that shit!? I have to acknowledge that horrible and humiliating feeling? That feels like death, admitting to that!* Of course, waking up to ourselves is a very individual process, and whatever your stance is on porn, it's important to start noticing where you may be breeding non-realities in your life. You may want to notice what porn brings up for you and what unmet needs are wanting to be known. If porn upsets you, ask yourself what is underneath those visceral feelings. From this mindset, porn becomes a simple foil; a pathway to self-knowledge.

Soul Reverb

Now that we've explored many different angles to broach the topic, it's time for reflection. Reach for your workbook or journal and write down your answers.

1. In what ways has porn played out in your life? In what ways has porn been helpful to you? And in what ways do you feel it has set you back?
2. What are the underlying needs you are trying to meet with porn? Do you have any unaddressed feelings that are being numbed by watching porn?
3. How comfortable are you with talking about your sexual needs and discomforts with your partner? What is blocking you from doing this?

Chapter Affirmations

- I have needs and I can express them.
- My dissatisfaction is always a symptom of a greater problem.
- To connect to others, I must first connect to myself.

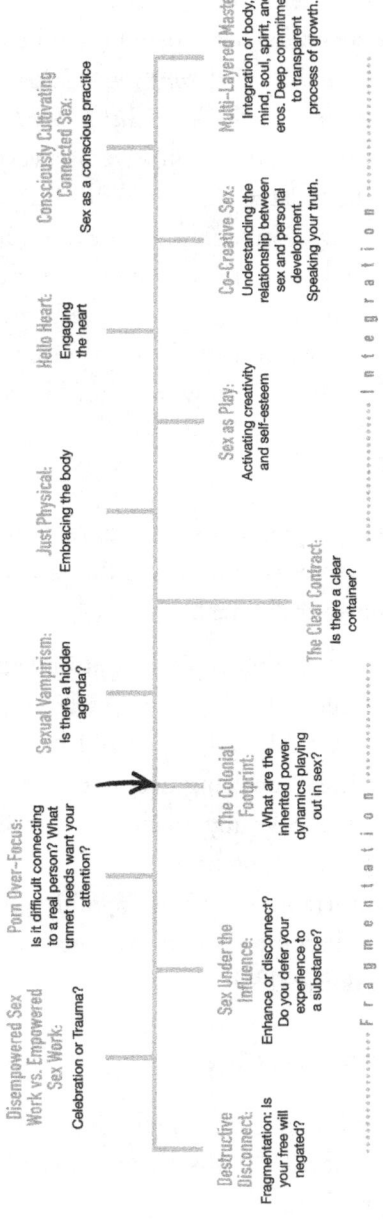

CHAPTER 5:

DECOLONIZE SEX

"First they ignore you, then they laugh at you, then they fight you, then you win."

—Mahatma Ghandi

Section 1. Outgrow Power Dynamics

Sex is an energetic exchange involving the very essence of who we are; this is why it is such an intimate transaction. We are sharing the energy, the very life force that moves through us. As it blasts through the core of our being, our sexual energy grazes and activates all the stored information held in our body. It wakes up everything, our pleasure, our shame, our past wounds, our inherited wounds, our entitlement and our unchecked fears. Our bodies remember everything—at least, until the memories are processed and released. Then, our bodies can finally let go of the past, meaning all those cellular memories of past wounding are finally evacuated and new possibilities and responses become available to us. But in a complex world bearing the marks of multiple layers of traumatic histories, there is a significant amount of unaddressed dynamics that are just waiting to be tended to. So what happens when you mix in the colonial footprint and unchecked power dynamics to sex?

Our sexual energy bears the imprint of all the baggage we inherited from our families growing up, our ancestral lines, our culture, our history—and even past lives, if you are willing to go there. What if that baggage involves widespread cultural trauma? What if that baggage comes with the message that "you are worth diddly squat" because of your economic or ethnic status? The ramifications of colonialism are far-reaching and at times so deeply ingrained in the status quo that they translate into systemic violence, which means it is hard to put your finger on the toxicity. It becomes an almost covert and erosive force that takes awakening to see.

These are the reasons why our discussion on sex and healing would be incomplete without addressing the colonial footprint.

Colonialism involves a foreign-imposed power structure of domination that deems some people valuable and others not. It is designed to bring political, social, economic, and more subtly, sexual advantages, to those holding the big end of the stick. For those unfamiliar with the colonial footprint, this would include the pain and anger that comes from racism, prejudice, injustice, loss of sovereignty, cultural depreciation, and cultural humiliation. When these issues remain unaddressed, they shape the everyday experience of large groups of people.

Colonial history, with imperialism as an economic subset to this, has impacted almost every piece of land and every group of people on Earth in some shape or form. No wonder this is a painful experience for so many. As we see with all dynamics, this plays out in the sexual realm. Sex is always a good barometer for what unspoken power dynamics are playing out in the world. This is why decolonizing sex is an essential step in healing sex in the world.

In this section you will:

- Identify the impact of colonial history on our sexual dynamics
- See how colonial practices affect dating patterns and certain ethnic groups
- Experience Devi Ward's story of healing the colonial footprint in her life
- Learn to free yourself from the impacts of colonial imprints
- Understand "decolonization" as a path to freedom

A Personal Note

I first became aware of colonialism when I was an idealistic teenager wanting to change the world. At a potluck/social justice meeting, with other inspired movers and shakers, I spotted a small, inconspicuous yet vibrant man from Mexico sashayed with a traditional woven garb sitting quietly on the sofa. It turned out that he was working on a master's thesis as an important cultural leader for the Otomi people. He was devising a proposal for a fourth-level government for indigenous people in Mexico. He was envisioning a new political order for the Mexican nation-state that empowered the indigenous people of the country, and was challenging the "Mestizo" blanket that was hiding away all the cultural diversity of the country.

When the Mexican government got wind of his ideas, they pulled away his financing, which left him sleeping on our common friend's couch. I was moved by his story and then decided to convince my mother to take him in, while he sent me down as an eighteen-year-old adventurer with a packsack to visit his family in San Pedro de Tultepec. This included a bucket list of other people to visit during my trip, including a Mayan priestess in Guatemala—who kicked started my personal healing journey.

Decolonize Sex

This got me thinking. What about the First Nations of my home country: Canada? Why hadn't I really learned about their history? And why had I never spoken to someone with this ancestry? At Trent University, there was a whole department devoted to First Nations, their history, their culture, the current-day politics and social realities. Most professors were First Nation people, while Iroquois, Ojibwe, Mi'kmaq, Innu and Inuit were amongst the enrolled student population. I had plenty to learn, to witness, and to digest.

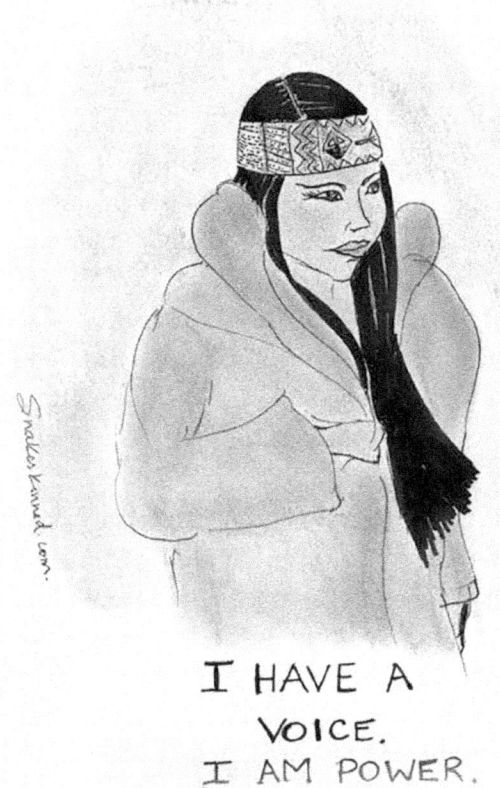

I HAVE A VOICE. I AM POWER.

But most notable was the friendship I created with my friend Vicki Proulx, a courageous Ojibwe-Oneida woman, Turtle Clan from her mother's lineage and Thunderbird Clan from her father's side. She and her sisters were very active in creating healing ceremonies, whether it be what they called at the time "unburdening" or via sweat lodges, they initiated me to the pain of colonialism.

As the burning sage wafted across the room, rattles shaking, drums resounding, their voices filled the room. There in front of my nineteen-year-old eyes, I would see them break down into tears and release all the pent-up pain. I would hear these pangs of pain run through my body. The pain of loss. The pain of betrayal. The pain of alienation. The pain of injustice. The unspeakable heartache. The pain of truth denied. The excruciating pain of seeing your community fall to pieces. Of seeing your culture devalued. To place this in time, this was unfolding six years before the publishing of "The Truth and Reconciliation Report" in Canada.

These ceremonies were deep purges from all the inherited toxic dynamics that had taken grip of their lives. They were courageously evacuating, one ceremony at a time, the colonial footprint from their lives. In this chapter, I will be talking about "decolonization" as a process of healing from historical, cultural, social, religious, and contextual trauma. It's the process of weeding out all the unhelpful beliefs that we inherited that do not serve our greatest outcome, and look at how these beliefs impact how sexuality plays out.

One of these painful ramifications was her brother's suicide in the wake of challenging a Jesuit priest who, assigned to her community, had sexually abused him. Being the Church's authority, he would sweep up the young boys of the community for weekends and the parents were expected to simply trust him, while he secretly abused them.

And yet my friends sat in circle, first chuckling and cracking jokes, often about sex, then in ceremony, crying, and puking their hearts out. Then laughing again. They were defining the very concept of decolonization for me. They were, one ceremony at a time, decolonizing 500 years of colonial rule that had disrupted their cultural identity and vibrancy. They were grieving all the disruption and pain that were widespread amongst their people, an echo that resounds around the world for many people.

Colonial forces have left wreckages of trauma across the globe. The footprint involves leaving behind significant clefts of inequality, whether it be economic, social, and, of course, sexual. Colonialism involves practices of imperialism, cultural genocide, slavery, and military interventions in the distant and not-so-distant past. The colonial principle organizes the world in ways that create important inequalities around resources, economic means and power. It decides who is valuable and who is not. Who is entitled, who isn't. Colonialism is about asserting power over a people and their land for economic gain, while eroding the vitality and sovereignty of their culture. An imposed domination structure often comes with "benefits," i.e. sexual acts of all kinds, that mirrors the established power dynamics.

Add Sex to the Mix

What happens to sex in places where there have been significant abuses? Where poverty is a by-product of colonial practices? What happens to the women? To the girls? To the boys? To the LGBT folk? For one, The Garden of Truth report[16] reveals that colonized people are overly represented in disempowered sex work. And what if we add in the tourist industry, poverty, and disposable cash? When people have been deemed "less valuable" through long-standing exploitative behaviors, whether it be slavery, cultural

---

16 http://www.prostitutionresearch.com/pdfs/Garden_of_Truth_Final_Project_WEB.pdf

genocide or military bullying, sex follows suit, and abuses of all grades start showing up.

Are You in the "Valuable Group?"

In fact, some groups get specifically targeted for various forms of sexual violence, murders, abuse and degrading behavior simply because they are deemed a vulnerable group. To be noted, "vulnerable" is a by-product of the erosive colonial practices. When the social structures break down, you become exposed. Also to be noted, systemic violence means people get away with it. This is what happens when you have been given a lesser status—people can get away with hurting you. Even killing you. This has become particularly apparent in the missing Aboriginal women crisis in Canada.

The heritage of colonial practices, imperialism, slavery and segregation leave deep clefts in the world and show up in various forms of exploitative sexual encounters, including "disempowered" sex work, human trafficking, which can appallingly even involve the police force—as was seen in Quebec.[17] It can also mean sending priests and nurs to communities when in fact they are known pedophiles and sexual predators hiding behind their authoritative frocks, protected by the church, and actions conveniently ignored by the state. These types of sexual transgressions enabled by colonial practices leave huge imprints on the sexual health and well-being of whole communities for generations if not dealt with.

Colonial Imprints and Dating Patterns

It also can show up in more subtle ways, such as dating patterns. People can be made to feel like they are worth less if they are of

---

17 https://globalnews.ca/news/2304898/allegations-police-abused-first-nations-women-in-val-dor-part-of-a-national-problem-observers-say/

this or that race. People may be rejected from coupling based on the color of their skin, their culture or their religion—and yes, this is still rampant today. It could be okay to "fuck" them, but not to date or marry them "officially." Or conversely, some cultures are sought out specifically to find submissive, demure wives because women are willing to do anything to escape the economic hardships of their country.

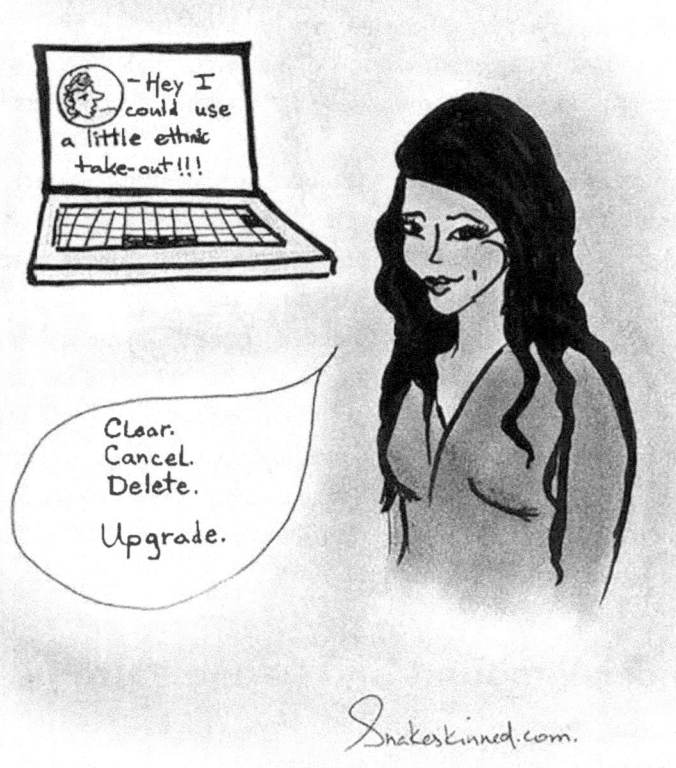

People have shared with me all kinds of racist attitudes that inform sexual behaviors, including comments such as these: "I could use a little ethnic takeout," said by a man to an East Indian woman in Vancouver on a dating app, or "I can't go out with you because of your skin color" said to a biracial American woman in Michigan to explain why a committed relationship was impossible. A Thai friend of mine sent me a social media post from an appalled peer of hers. The young woman was disgusted by a comment that had been addressed to her white male friend of many years as they had entered a nightclub together: "Is she your weekend girlfriend? Keep on enjoying the Bangkok life, dude!"

These comments may not be so surprising in the context of the colonial footprint. Lots of shit went down in history! And until addressed thoroughly, until we work through the power dynamics and prejudices that we've inherited, entitlement and poor self-worth continue to ravage the world.

Jet-Set Sexual Entitlement

It is sad to say that people actually travel the world because they know they can get away with certain sexual behaviors that would not be acceptable back in their home country. Furthermore, there are vast financial inequalities wedged into these dynamics. Some people travel to certain destinations because women are viewed as "easy," "submissive," having "tight pussies," "less valuable," "promiscuous" or "less protected" by their culture and legal structures. Or they go places where children or the LGTQ community are not protected, or targeted because they are vulnerable and at risk. The underlying issue of poverty exposes many to awful treatment.

I've heard people gloat that "if you go there, you can get whatever you want, no questions asked." This exploits their position of entitlement. It is especially revealing that they would not behave in such a way back home, right? Listen up—this is the colonial footprint at work.

Besides lacking basic human decency, such behaviors inflict another layer of disempowerment and disconnection in sex. How can sex be truly good for both parties if the act involves taking advantage of someone and banking on their weaknesses or their economic destitution? Or conversely, how can you enjoy sex if you feel less worthy than your partner? If you think, *I am treated like crap in this relationship, but it's better than nothing...* how about considering again. Who made you believe that? What are you actually worth? How can you reclaim your inherent human right to dignity?

As seen with my First Nation's friends' deep commitment to healing, the good news is that we can free ourselves of such nasty dynamics. Who wants to go around carrying shame for the color of one's skin even for another day? Who wants to feel eternally disempowered because of colonial history, playing out one's damaged self-worth in sexual encounters, or be treated like crap for no apparent reason? Who wants to let an entitled person dictate their worth? Who wants to live life angry all the time? Well, you can if you want to, of course—we are free human beings, after all—but as the ego of your life, you have a choice. Instead of merely existing or barely surviving, wouldn't you rather start living an empowered life?

Although anger is a necessary emotion in response to injustice, to remain attached to anger also keeps you in a state of fragmentation. Disempowerment stays glued to your skin.

This is why up levelling your sense of self-worth and the quality of sex in your life involves releasing all those damaging belief systems and emotions. They are the by-product of lies. If we consider that real power only comes from within, through accessing one's fullest expression of humanity, through embodying inner freedom, by becoming a fully integrated person, it is interesting to see that colonial power is only possible when snatching power from someone else; they become powerful only because they take power away from other people. It is not the result of them accessing their own integrated power from wholeness.

Let's see the colonial footprint in action as it plays out for the international sex educator Devi Ward as she frees herself from the colonial footprint.

Devi Ward's Story—Decolonize Cellular Memory

I initially got to know Devi Ward as an international sex educator and Tantra teacher, of Tibetan lineage, who guided me over the course of a few months. Then she agreed to share her stories of trauma and healing as a biracial woman growing up in a white American world. At the end of this interview process, I offered her a session in my modality of healing—The Akashic Records—which allows me to create a sacred container for my clients and support them in finding stubborn patterns that hold them back. From there, they can free themselves of whatever is causing the issue to reoccur.

Devi's story involves growing up amidst racial slurs. Starting quite young, she began to experience discrimination, disrespect, and focused negativity for her mere existence. This became clear when her first-grade crush had told her that "She was so fucking ugly, that when she died, he wanted to burn all that frizzy nigger hair off her head and pour acid all over her ugly nigger face so no one would ever have to hurt their eyes looking at her again."[18]

---

[18] In recounting her story, Devi Ward explicitly requested that these insults not be edited out or softened to fully capture the offensive nature of these experiences.

She was confused. This barrage of insults had followed a simple declaration of love to him.

Things intensified when she moved to Michigan where her family ended up living down the street from the KKK grand dragon. She recalls regular harassment—being called out, hissed and spit at, simply for being bi-racial. One day when she was coming home from school, three boys accosted Devi. One of them barked at her, "Don't let me catch you alone, nigger! You ugly, fake, half-breed nigger. I will cut off your head and throw your ugly nigger body in a ditch." From this, she started to think something must be blatantly wrong with her.

Another important imprint came from her father himself. He was a brilliant black man—one of the first fighter jet pilots in Michigan, who had learned to speak Japanese fluently, and who was a techie before tech was the norm. Immediately after reading his resumé, employers would call him in for an interview. However, upon arrival and the realization of his skin color, all enthusiasm would evaporate.

With no healthy outlet for this systematic injustice and violence, her father grew tremendously angry and would take it out on his family. One night, Devi witnessed her black father holding her white mother against the wall and pouring grape juice over her head. That night, her mother packed up their suitcases and left with Devi and her brother in the middle of the night.

Regardless, Devi loved her father dearly and always yearned for a strong father/daughter connection, in part because she now only saw hers periodically. She admired him tremendously and cherished their deep conversations. So when his violence erupted the household, it always caught her off-guard and deeply hurt her.

One day while she was staying with him, she had come home from parading her new short-shorts in public and was delighted to get some honks from passersby. But when she got home, her father was waiting in a fit of rage. Someone had stained his immaculate white carpets. As soon as Devi entered the front door, he pounced on her and pinned her to the ground. He proceeded to whip her with his metal belt, then held her neck with his two hands, almost choking her to death. Somehow, she found the strength to say, "If you kill me, my ghost will come back and kill you in your sleep!" Suddenly, he broke out of his angered trance, left her lying on the floor gasping, and without a response, walked upstairs.

These traumas accumulated and played themselves out in various ways throughout her life. For one thing, she grew up believing that because of her skin color, she was second class for dating and sex. She could be the brown sugar on the side, but not the official girlfriend. She could be a groupie, but never the trophy girlfriend. Later when she became a stripper, she felt second class to the white strippers. And many times, her lovers would abandon her for the privileged and educated white woman. This left a deep cleft in her heart and eroded her sense of self-worth.

But even stranger "colonial" dynamics started playing out. She describes entering a home in Hawaii as the housekeeper to a very wealthy spiritual new-age guru. As the dynamics played out, she became what she describes as their "house nigger." They were taking advantage of her time and expecting her to be the full-time maid without compensation, as opposed to their hired cleaning lady on a specific schedule. Overnights often occurred since apparently the wife had become overwhelmed after childbirth. Devi was expected to be tirelessly at their beck and call, and she had trouble refusing their requests.

When sleeping over in their mansion, she started having the most peculiar and disturbing dreams. In her dreams, she would be energetically pulled into the master bedroom and invited to have sex with them, without feeling she could resist any demands. On occasion, a friend of hers also spent the night. When Devi spoke about the strange dreams, they eerily learned that both shared almost exactly the same dream, frame-by-frame. This was very odd and disconcerting. The spiritual guru in the couple did give off this creepy sexualized vibe that felt off-putting and invasive.

But it didn't end there. One time after she slept the night, she discovered bruises in her inner thigh, like injuries from sex. She had no recollection of hurting herself in any way. Nothing could explain the sudden presence of bruises in that intimate place. This was a most peculiar happening. Had she been drugged during the night and covertly abused? Was he practicing some form of non-consensual astral travel during the night and violating her energetic boundaries? She could not figure it out.

Whatever it was, something had happened, and she felt violated. When considering the colonial heritage of power dynamics and the ensuing sexual violence that accompanied it, whether it be via a plantation master raping the female "slave labor" under gunpoint or imposing sexual favors on the "maid" of the house, a.k.a. raping her, these were commonplace by-products of slavery, in all its ramifications and permutations.

When Devi finally discovered the healing capacity of tantra, she felt like she was releasing generations of colonial pain. During her tantra sessions, she would break down in sobs, screaming, and crying out all the pain and trauma she had collected as a biracial woman in a white world. It was the first time she started understanding where all the pain had come from, what she had been carrying and fighting against, unconsciously, all her life. The process felt like going through hell, and yet it allowed her to experience deep relief, and even high, sublime states of bliss.

At the end of our interview process, it just so happened that we were both in Vancouver and we could finally meet, which we did over some Indian cuisine. She was very excited to introduce me to her newlywed love. When she arrived, she was elated: it was the first time in her life she felt so satisfied on all levels with a man. This tall, handsome, bright, kind white man really knew how to love her deeply. The thing she had been wanting and searching for all her life finally was here in full flesh and form. And she could actually have it.

But her "decolonizing" process did not end there, which is not surprising when you consider that healing happens in layers. Racism can be deeply traumatizing, and subtle issues and beliefs get passed down the ancestral line without our awareness. Devi was telling me about her Authentic Tantra business over supper and how she was experiencing technological glitches as they were getting ready for their launch. This wasn't the first time she'd complained about such glitches.

I commented on the recurrence. Patterns always point to the root of a dynamic. In our session, some very interesting things transpired. The pattern was a replay from her father. Every time he was ready to land an amazing new job, he would be turned down upon being seen. Every time Devi wanted to upscale, some form of self-sabotaging energy would appear.

When we dug a little deeper, we discovered that behind all these technological glitches was the anger she had inherited from her father. Now it was getting in the way of her accomplishing her goals. Regardless, she wasn't sure she wanted to let go of her anger, as it energized her to fight for equality.

The message I was getting: "She has every right in the world to be angry, but if she wants to get to another level, both in her business and in her spiritual practice as a tantra teacher, she has to let go of anger." This was a profound realization for Devi. And even if it was somewhat hard to digest, she understood it perfectly. It was clear that anger had its place in the world, but that Devi's capacity to transmute that anger would in fact be a much more powerful gift for humanity. Her transformation would be a potent medicine for the masses, far greater than what her anger was capable of. Within the sacred space of the Akashic Records, we started releasing all belief systems that no longer served her.

Decolonize Sex

A week later, Devi told me that after our session, some intense things unfolded. The session had catalyzed a profound purging and purification for her. The night after, she had dreamt that she was raging around trying to choke people. While choking people, she would experience a deep sense of gratification and release because she was giving away the anger. When her father had choked her, almost to death, he had potently transferred his feelings of failure, injustice, and racial pain to her. He was giving her an energetic transmission that would imprint itself onto her psyche and into her body.

Then the next night, out of the blue, her throat started to hurt and within an hour she felt like hands were holding her neck and exerting a tightening pressure. A fever then overtook her body. And to top it off, the next morning, she coughed up a burr-like brown, hardened clump stuck at the back of her throat. She thought, *what the fuck is this* !? She couldn't believe it. It looked like a fat, hairy spider.

Subsequently, tangible life results started rolling in. At the beginning of our session, she had asked for the removal of any blocks impeding the success of her brand. Thereafter, Devi's new clarity showed her that the current brand representative had been leading them in the wrong direction. They decided to renegotiate the contract, but instead, the person quit. After his departure, they discovered how sloppy the work had been and how detrimental to the business it would have been in the long run. Not only did she celebrate the fact that it was a peaceful dissolution, but it also made room for new members to join the team that were 100% behind their brand.

Devi's story not only illustrates the ramifications of racism and colonialism, but it also shows how poison can be transformed into powerful medicine. Devi's story models the process of decolonization, meaning healing from deep historical and societal trauma in her signature powerful way. It also means stopping the passing on of this "angry" hot potato through a very powerful process of deactivation. When you really look into this type of healing, the prospect of this kind of courage is incredibly significant for our collective future.

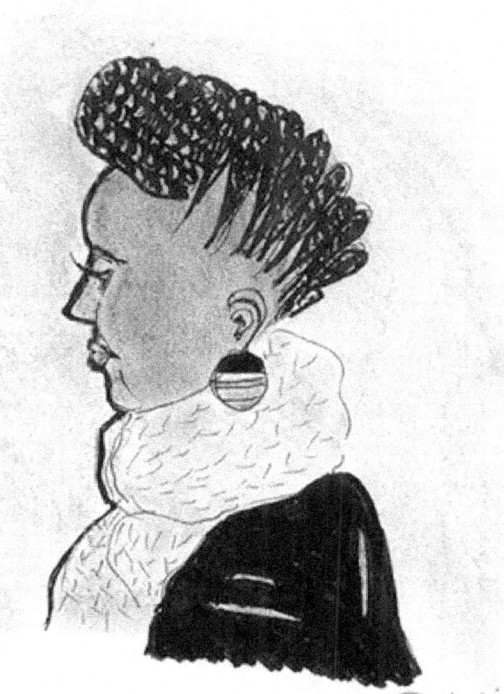

I AM BEAUTY.
I AM POWER.

How Do We Get Relief?

The path to relief is finding where the core of our self-worth issues lie: where did we start believing that our culture, ethnicity or race was worth less than any other? Who made us feel that way? How did we over-compensate for this misguided belief? When did we take that belief on?

This also includes shifting out of a scarcity mindset. "I can only get this, so…" "This is my only chance at improving my economic situation, so…", "Who else is going to want me…" "This is my only chance to…", "This is all I can do to survive…", "I've always been treated this way, so…"

These power dynamics and beliefs impact how we relate to one another and limit what is possible for us. They show up in sex in how we value ourselves and our self-worth, what we think we can get and not get, what we endure, what we tolerate, what we think we deserve or don't deserve.

Becoming fully conscious of these dynamics and naming them is half the battle. The next step, if you are willing and able, is to release these beliefs from your body. Our worth comes from the inside, not from the outside, even if we can get distracted in believing otherwise. If you are ready to take the leap, it's time to say no to carrying crap around that doesn't belong to you. It's time for your empowered self to show up and enjoy good, wholesome sex from that empowered rock star place and feel the greatness of who you are.

This is the process of decolonizing sex: freeing oneself of all those lies that are slowly chipping away at your self-worth. Decolonizing sex is a very sacred process that starts with ourselves, and it keeps on going and going and going, way beyond ethnicity and race, until freedom is experienced on all levels of our being.

It's a truly profound experience that starts with sex, but when you get the hang of it, it starts decolonizing your entire soul.

Bob definitely had it right: it's time to "free yourself of mental slavery!"

Soul Reverb

Now that you've considered the colonial footprint, it's time for reflection. Reach for your journal or workbook and answer these questions.

1. What traces of colonialism can you find in your life? How does it impact you? What kinds of power dynamics show up in your life?
2. Can you identify where your self-worth has suffered? In what ways? Has entitlement been an issue in your life? How does "guilt" disempower you?
3. How have these beliefs limited your life: what you think you deserve or not, what you think you need to endure/or tolerate, what you think you can get or not?
4. How have these dynamics played out in sexuality? How has it shown up in your ancestral lineage?

Section Affirmations

- When I am angry, it's only the tip of the iceberg.
- When I process my pain, I gain power.
- When I release my pain, I experience freedom.

Section 2. Beyond Orientation

Now, let's decolonize beyond culture and race, and bring that same principle to sexual orientation.

In this section you will:

- Identify the impact of cultural and religious programming on sexual orientation
- Experience Hasina Juma's struggle to understand her sexual orientation
- Learn about the pains of denying sexual orientation
- Witness Hasina's enlightened process to coming out
- Appreciate the freedom and power with owning sexuality

As my Six Nations Mohawk friend and founder of "Ka'nikonhriyohtshera: Fostering Emergence of the Good Mind" Diane Hill has said, "Once you start the process of decolonization, you should keep on going, and it requires a conscious choice to do so." To be successful in freeing yourself, as in the case of Devi, decolonization must become a principle to live by. According to Diane, this is the mindset to adopt: "I am choosing to decolonize my mind of any 'foreign' negative or limiting belief that is not in alignment with my true essence, which is an unconditionally loving spirit."

Diane explains that the colonization of your mind is a very subtle process that happens over time. "It can start at the moment of conception, through birth, and as you grow into adulthood, throughout your entire lifecycle, until you start noticing that something is off or wrong, meaning that you start to question both who and what you really are." When you take decolonizing into the spiritual realm, it means "bringing to the surface any misaligned beliefs that disassociate you from a sense of being true to yourself or what you consider to be your personal truth, which means how you perceive yourself." Thus, decolonizing takes place in layers. You keep peeling back the layers of misaligned beliefs that have become embedded into you as memories.

Decolonization allows you to consciously weed out anything that is in the way of expressing and realizing your essence. It's the process of reclaiming those areas that have been overshadowed by shame. Reclaiming yourself puts you back on the path of true freedom. Decolonization is an inner job, a path to inner freedom, that then radiates out into society, helping to reshape it in a more wholesome way.

Shame as Correction Officer

One day as I was gleaning the internet, I haphazardly fell onto a YouTube video on the theme of overcoming shame by the internet "mystic" sensation Teal Swan. Her description of shame rang so true in my soul. She explained that shame is the painful feeling of comparing yourself to your own adopted standards and then falling short of them.

Essentially, we are born within a family, within a culture, that has social and cultural values. When children contradict or transgress the threshold of these values, they are punished, reprimanded or simply disapproved of. The children go on to adopt these cultural and social values for themselves in order to be loved and feel a sense of belonging. The less awakened a society, the more invasive the socialization process is.

As children, we much rather adopt these values than experience the pain of disapproval and embarrassment of rejection, or worse, the ominous threat of ostracization, which touches the very core of our instinct to survive. Swan explains that we go on to internalize these belief systems and become our very own corrections officer, which is less painful than being policed by someone else. Shame takes over to avoid future negative consequences.

So how can you emancipate from shame? By decolonizing your mind from all your false beliefs that inhibit you from simply being "YOU" in your fullest integrity. It is the ultimate state of flow where you don't need to repress any part of yourself—a sure sign: you become fully self-expressed! Unease and shame will show you where those misaligned beliefs are. The process of decolonizing allows you to address the glitch or the dissonance happening between your adopted values, or the values that were shoved onto you and reassert the legitimacy of your own natural identity and its inherent worth.

Cheers to that! Our sexual expression and identity is obviously at the core of this uncovering; how could it be otherwise? It's the very life force that moves through us. When we don't respect this life force, we operate from a suboptimal state.

Individuation as Courage

To fully own who you are is an act of courage, through and through. Individuation means becoming yourself fully. It means getting out of flock mentality and making space for your true self, which for many can be quite daunting and almost always involves growing pains. It's the courageous act of normalizing what has previously been deemed "abnormal." And you achieve this by owning yourself and making room for more possibilities. Well, we are infinitely creative beings, aren't we? We are constantly generating more potential with our creativity, our imaginations, and re-imaginations. Whole societies shift because of these collective re-imaginings, which in turn is sparked by someone's individual reimagination.

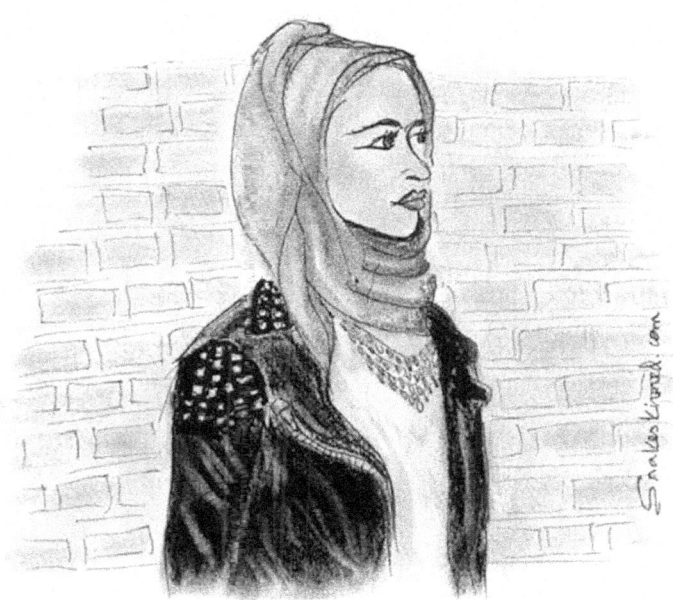

I AM MY OWN POWER.

This also involves butting up against resistance. People can't always tolerate change in others because it challenges them to reflect, wake up to a certain reality, and become aware of what they might need to look at, own, accept and even change in their lives. Usually, they resist change because of some permutation of fear. To carve out space for your unique identity when it has not previously been recognized or valued by your community is a powerful act of reclamation. What is more powerful than fully owning your truth?

So let's dive into Hasina Juma's story about reclaiming her sexual identity against a backdrop of a tight-knit religious community and strong cultural socialization.

Hasina Juma's Story—On Religion, Orientation, and Sex

Hasima Juma's story is a testimony to the importance of the courageous process of reclamation. She has been bravely carving out space for her sexual identity when it seemed at complete odds with the core values of her community, and in the process she is creating space for others too.

A second-generation Canadian of South Asian descent, Hasina was born to a Muslim family in the small prairie city of Saskatoon. Her family had previously settled in Tanzania and had lived there over the course of two generations. But when the political climate in Uganda and other neighboring countries started shifting drastically by expelling the South Asian community out of their country, Hasina's parents decided to pre-emptively relocate, first to England, then to Canada.

After her birth, they relocated in the 80s to a middle-class suburban town in the vicinity of Edmonton. Everything about Hasina seemed at odds with her predominantly white, mostly Protestant, middle-class Edmonton neighborhood: she was person of color of African and South Asian lineage and she was Muslim. As Hasina tried to piece together who she was, her family's origins, what her religious beliefs were, and navigated spoken and unspoken codes of conducts, she remembers spending most of her childhood trying to resolve this question: "how do I explain my identity to people?" This was a question that would take on a whole new dimension when her sexual identity would surface later. Hasina often grappled with the feeling that people didn't understand her.

Growing up, her religious community was very tight, and that is where she would spend most of her time outside of school. There was the prayer center, then there were the many social and religious functions and celebrations, and she was part of their popular ball-hockey league. It was with this community that

Hasina felt most at home and spiritually nourished. She describes her upbringing as good. Her religious community taught her to be very ambitious, to have goals, and to go for them.

She describes herself as being the product of a very open Canadian culture infused with pop culture, tv and music videos, combined with a conservative element that came from her religion. Sexuality was a private affair; you discussed it in the home, and even then, it was private. She doesn't recall ever having an open conversation about sexuality, nor love, with her parents. In grade 6, they had basic sex-ed at school, but that was it.

She had to learn about sexuality from the outside, because, for one, there was an intergenerational pattern of repressing sexuality in her family: sex was intended for procreation. Nothing else was spoken of nor encouraged. There was no talk about the positive empowerment of sex. And to be fair, her parents were never taught about sex either, so when it came to her, well, she ended up just suppressing it too. Sex is dangerous. Sex is bad. Just wearing a tank top was showing too much skin. In her environment, it became clear that sexuality was not embraced, and even less so in a holistic way. This resulted in her repressing her own sexuality and sexual orientation for the greater part of her life.

There was no clear moment when Hasina realized, "OMG, I'm bisexual." She feels like she was born like that, but it was so deeply hidden away that it only started appearing when she was willing and able to see it. A series of events during her undergraduate degree and afterwards just kept on creeping up on her. Those were the years when many people started getting married, and she would attend their weddings. She would notice the attractive men, but she would also notice the women.

"It wasn't: 'Oh, she is so pretty and wearing a pretty dress.' It was: 'OMG, she is so gorgeous and I'm having butterflies going on inside myself.' And I wished I could go and talk to her." But she always had this relentless feeling inhibiting her. "I'm at a religious South Asian wedding, no one can find out." In fact, one time she blurted out how attractive a woman was to her, but then quickly had to retract it and reframe it to make it acceptable. She immediately watered down the intensity by saying that she was attractive when what she really wanted to say was "I find you really attractive."

She also noticed that her friends, the majority of whom were women, were affectionate amongst themselves, but she seemed to have stronger feelings than her friends and would often attach things to it when they wouldn't. Whenever she would go to hang out with her friends, and they would talk about the hot guys, or their celebrity crushes, she always felt like she was biting her tongue, which gave her a deadening feeling. People around her always asked her why she wasn't married yet. "Like, what are your criteria, Hasina?" Or, "Where's your boyfriend Hasina?" Secretly, Hasina always wanted to change the word "boyfriend" to "partner," but again, she couldn't bring herself to say it.

Even if she was starting to notice her feelings, it was hard to fully embrace them. At university, she would socialize with the members of her religious community and they were all straight. They were all striving to get degrees, be the best in their careers. She didn't know anyone that was Canadian, that was a person of color, from her religious community, and that was "out" and thriving. She concluded by de facto that it mustn't be safe coming out.

There were, of course, university associations that could help her, but seeing she was so engrossed in her own community where no one was openly part of the LGBTQ2+ community, in addition to the fact that there was a belief in her community that you don't ask for help because that is a sure sign of weakness, reaching out to the LGBTQ2+ associations didn't even dawn on her. And of course, if she did come out, the consequences were unknown: would she be disowned by her family? Would her family be discriminated against in her religious community? Would she lose the community she grew up in? Instead, she decided, "I am just going to hide my identity."

Furthermore, Hasina had trouble trusting her feelings. She describes herself as having a very masculine approach at the time; she needed "proof" that this was indeed what was going on for her. She already knew she was attracted to men, but she needed to confirm her attraction to women. Yet by the time she reached university, the easiest route seemed to simply repress her sexual nature all together. She focused all her attention on getting that piece of paper and the idea of traveling the world.

This urge to figure out if she was interested in women followed her—relentlessly. But how could she confirm this? She couldn't go to the bar; what if she saw someone she knew? That would just be awkward, she concluded. And then how do you ask? And what about this whole "hook-up" thing; was that the way? How do you find someone that's not straight!? She concluded: "I don't even know how to navigate these conversations!" And yet, that person appeared in her life and it was confirmed. She finally proved it to herself: she was into women.

But still, there was no way anyone could find out about it.

It had been ten years since she had adopted this dual persona. In July 2015, her world became very dark: she hit her rock-bottom moment and thought, *if I don't change the way I'm operating, I'm not going to survive.*

That is when she sought out a way she could start accepting her sexual orientation. At that point she still had a very masculine approach to life, i.e. "give me a problem and I will "solve it." She says, "I was very ambitious. But what are my feelings? What are "feelings"? How do I communicate feelings without taking myself out?" She put herself through counselling, which she did online secretly from her bedroom. She didn't want her parents to find out: going for counselling in her community was taboo. She found someone in Vancouver that was part of her ethnic community and religious affiliation, and to top that off, a professional psychotherapist. Hasina called her and said, "Listen, I need to come out." Hasina was under the impression that the psychotherapist would give her the ten easy steps to follow and then she could just come out.

It wasn't that simple. First she had to reconnect to her feelings—repressed for so many years—and learn to communicate them. At first, this greatly irritated her. She wondered why they were always foraging stuff back from her childhood. "That was a foreign concept to me. I was like, what was going on when I was six does not have an impact on my life now." But as Hasina followed the process, things started clicking into place. She learned what it meant to "process" her emotions, which was not the easiest situation since she was living in her parents' home. All the surges of emotions she would have, and the need to process them, had to remain incognito to anyone outside her bedroom door.

Her parents started wondering why she was isolating herself like that and said, "You are always in your room, you come back from abroad and disown us. You don't interact with us!" But it wasn't that simple for her. "I had come back to Edmonton to search for a job, and yet I had all these feelings inside of myself. My world was really dark; if I don't get help now, something was going to happen. Something was not going to end well."

The darkness came from this feeling that all her relationships were somewhat fake because she couldn't truly be herself. She felt a lot of shame about who she was. At times she would lash out at her family members because she had so much unspoken anger. "Why are you always on me!" She would deflect or make things worse. She wasn't arguing for that individual situation. "Actually," she says, "I was angry at myself. I didn't have the courage to come out. It was a lot of projection because I wasn't owning my responsibility."

Yet at one point, this double life had overtaken her whole body and she couldn't function anymore. In addition, intimate relationships were not working out and she couldn't speak freely about it. She couldn't express to anyone what was upsetting her. Her whole interface with the world felt contrived. She was not going for her dreams because she had this lingering feeling of never being enough. It didn't matter if she had just graduated with a double masters in Europe, that she was at the top of her class; she just couldn't access any feelings of happiness. She was at a loss on how to cultivate it. "How do I get to that inner happiness that is unlimited," she wondered. "Something is not right, here. I want to tell people who I am, but I don't have the courage to tell them. What if I am rejected? What if they don't understand me? I am going to be alone."

As she dove deeper into counselling, she also started participating in personal growth workshops that were shedding light on so many topics she was grappling with, such as self-worth, empowerment and self-nurturing. These workshops were revolutionary for Hasina. But they also compounded this dual life. Whenever there were events happening in her religious community, she couldn't explain why she wasn't attending; she always felt at a loss for words and justifications. She could never fully own why she was doing what she was doing.

There is also an added layer embedded in the South Asian community: "If I do something to gain my parents' approval, I am okay. If I do something that they don't approve of, then in South Asian culture it is very common that you feel, OMG, this can't be right." Hasina recognized how difficult it was to then trust herself and her own needs. The expectation of attending family and religious function would weigh heavily on her. There was also the people-pleasing aspect. "You see, you never share your personal issues, you always have to portray this image that everything is 'alright', even if it isn't. The difficult stuff stays in the house. I had to break with all that. I can make choices for myself that make sense to me."

The counselling work and workshops were essential to her coming out. They allowed her to do all the foundational work so she could feel solid the day it would happen. It was only in retrospect that she realized how important that initial phase was. Once it was covered, they started talking "coming out" and what that would actually look like.

The day she came out, she had her parents sitting in front of her and her brother was on the phone. Hasina recognized that all her previous work allowed her to show up from a loving and grounded space. It allowed her to express "I am sharing this with you because it is part of who I am," rather than, "I am a bisexual, OMG, and I am going to run out the door now!" It allowed her to come from a very different place.

It is clear to Hasina that if she had done it the other way, there would have been a much higher chance that it wouldn't have been received on the other side. "So when I came out, I explained what it is to be bisexual. A bisexual is when I love someone, I look at their soul and the gender doesn't really matter." She also explained why she had kept the secret for so long. In that conversation, her father explained that he grew up in a country where the LGBTQ2+ community was not openly present. "I haven't grown up with this, but as a family, we are here to support you. We are willing to learn." And then he said, "How can we support you?"

"When I was preparing, I didn't know what the reactions could be, because on the one hand you could have your parents disown you, or they can say they love you, or it can be somewhere in between." So when her father said that, she was dumbfounded. All she could find to say was, "I don't know how to answer that question, let me get back to you." This moment was profound for Hasina. "For me, it was really big. They may not have understood where I was coming from, but they loved me regardless. This is really huge because when your blood family accepts you, you know that if you come out somewhere else, in front of colleagues, friends, extended family, you know at least that your immediate family loves you. If they didn't support me, it would have been a double whammy."

She gave them time to digest the news. She knew they would have their own process of coming out. She knew that other courageous conversations would need to be had. While she was going through her coming out, she needed to also be there for them since they were taking in and digesting the information—questions and fears would most probably surface. She had to balance all these things. The next step would be to announce it to the extended family.

Her family still wondered: "Why do you need to tell the whole extended family? Isn't it a private affair?" Hasina had enough of hiding, shutting parts of herself down or doing contortion acts to avoid speaking about her sexual identification. She wanted to have space to be free, to be transparent with what was going on for her with all the people in her life, which included her family. "I didn't want to talk about my sexual orientation in every conversation, but I just wanted to be me where I didn't have to filter what I was saying. This would give me the freedom to chat about the good things happening in my life, the challenging ones, share cool stories I saw on the news about LGBTQ2+ or simply share my hopes and dreams without filtering information."

She wanted to reclaim the space and normalcy of who she is and how she identifies, so she drafted a letter and told them, "Before I share with you, I just want to say that I am still the same person and the one piece that you do know about me, well, you'll just know a little bit more now." She then explained how she identifies and, using her background in communications, she proceeded to answer all the questions she thought they would be curious about, saying, "I have known this for ten years, but I kept it to myself, but now I feel it is the time to share this to have a much more honest conversation." To her surprise, her extended family reached back out to her and affirmed that this news didn't change their relationship to her and that they loved her just as much. This meant the world to Hasina, as family is really important to her.

The next thing she had to sort out on her journey was where she belonged and where she didn't belong. She explains that when you are in the closet, you are so used to compromising yourself to make everyone else comfortable. "So, when you are out, there is this whole thing of owning who you are. It's an awkward feeling." But this is an essential piece. With this renewed commitment to authenticity and transparency, she quickly became aware of the spaces where she felt comfortable and the spaces where she didn't.

One of the uncomfortable places was her religious community. This was deeply painful to Hasina. This space had been part of her for thirty years. It was not just a prayer center, the place where you connect to God, but it was also what gave her a sense of belonging and community. This baffled her. "What do you replace that with?" she wondered. There was no how-to guide for that.

She tried getting her mind around what seemed like profound contradictions: "I am Canadian, and I am accepted, yet in my ethnic community, I am basically invisible." She explains that there is this perception in the South Asian community that LGTBQ2+ happens in Canadian society, but that it doesn't happen in their community, and even less so in her religious community. This is probably the case in other religious communities as well, whether you are Jewish, Catholic, or Protestant. She wondered, "how do I disentangle this?" She also wondered how she was going to nourish her spiritual yearning and re-create an authentic community for herself.

It was most painful when religious celebrations were observed in her community because she would have this yearning to be part of it. But if she no longer felt safe and fully accepted for who she was, how could she enjoy it? It wasn't that she was overtly disrespected in her religious community; it was more a feeling of dissonance. When she would be in prostration at the prayer hall, instead of feeling the peace she had once felt, it was replaced by this feeling of hollowness and frustration. "My frustration is that everyone has a soul and it doesn't have a gender label on it. So then why over the centuries have we misinterpreted scripts? We have created structures that have excluded people, and this is not only the case for Muslims, it's the case across all faiths. No one has been able to crack this paradox."

She decided to no longer go to the prayer center, nor attend social functions, because she just couldn't quell the conflict in her soul. She couldn't get that sense of fulfillment she was looking for. Instead, it would awaken this internal turmoil. "Here, LGBTQ2+ are not considered, which makes me basically invisible, so why am I doing this?" She started debating the question *am I religious or am I simply spiritual?*

She continued to work on herself, embodying her sexuality, and it started becoming clear that the more she would integrate her sexual energy and embrace it, the more she would notice how all spheres of her life were transforming. Her family started noticing news articles on the LGBTQ2+ community in mainstream media and collecting them for her. It also sparked engaging discussions around the dinner table. On a personal level, she noticed that by owning her sexual energy, she was also liberating her creative energy. The more she felt like she was finding her voice and her power center, the ripple effects on her life became beyond what she had initially imagined.

Suddenly, her life purpose started coming into focus; she created a platform to carve out more space and understanding for bisexual people of color and their families, which could also be relevant to people of color under the larger umbrella of LGBTQ2+. Her platform sets out to support both individuals coming out and their families. Hasina Juma is stepping up, while newspaper articles, social media lives, political networking, and speaking gigs are lining up to catapult her message to new heights.

Hasina's introspective journey and commitment to processing her pain has given her this unshakable power that is trailblazing a vaster understanding of the intersection between sexual identification, people of color, and the soul. And to top this off, a few months after we spoke, she officially shared on social media that she was in love! All that work on consolidating who she truly was finally paid off with the gift of an amazing and inspiring partner. Keep your eyes peeled on this rising leader and influencer.

This story shows us Hasina's process of undoing all the inherited belief systems that were getting in the way of her expressing her true authentic sexual energy. It is a testimony to how deep this process can go. Yes, our inherited religious dogmas, cultural constructs, and our family values can actually negate the very thing we are. That is why decolonizing is so powerful. Who we are is defined in an inside-out process, which is the true process of individuation.

And what's more, retrieving the various levels of your being means that what is meant to be you can come back into wholeness for you. Misguided ideas, constructs, and dogmas ultimately fragment us from our true essence, and this is where pain comes in. Who wants to be alienated from their true essence? With this story, we see how powerful ideas and frames of mind had disconnected Hasina from an important part of her being: her sexuality.

Here is an individual on the front lines of reclaiming space for difference and safe expression. Considering how difficult this is for so many people, it is thrilling to see individuals step up and own themselves.

Now that you've explored another layer of decolonizing, it's time for reflection.

1. Where has this broader concept of colonialism affected your identity? What values have you adopted that ultimately negate the essence of who you are?
2. In what ways do you withhold your true identity? How does it affect your sexual expression?
3. What messages have you received about your sexuality or other parts of yourself that make it unsafe for you to truly be self-expressed, both sexually and beyond?

Section Affirmations

- When I hide who I am, I hurt myself.
- I am not who my parents tell me to be. I am my own powerful person.
- When I own myself, I experience freedom.
- When I speak my truth, I am freedom.

Decolonize Sex

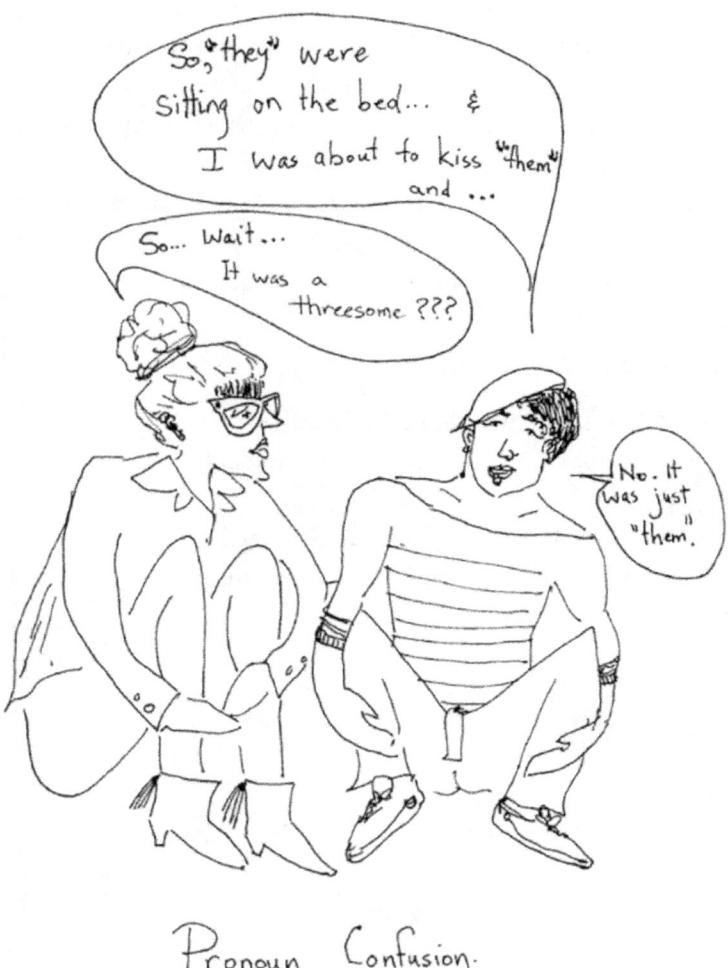

Pronoun Confusion.

Section 3. Expand Gender

Now, let's take this concept of decolonizing one step further. What happens when your body and gender don't feel in alignment with your essence? What if the glove you've been given is not the right shape for your hand? To bring this into alignment is another deep and challenging process that requires a lot of courage. This is the story of someone who found peace and equanimity in undergoing a sex change.

Let's dive into Sarah's story of sexual reassignment to find true inner alignment and peace of mind, from he to she: one step further in aligning the outside with the inside.

In this section you will:

- Learn about the process, the reasons, the challenges, the conditions of gender reassignment
- Learn about overcoming resistance and the experience of community

Sarah's Story—Gender Reassignment

I had a chance to talk to Sarah about her physical transition just eight weeks after her gender reassignment operation. She is twenty-seven now, but already knew at the age of nineteen that she wanted to go through with the physical transition from male to female. She just knew she needed to be a little more mature before making it happen; she needed time to ensure she was making the correct decision for herself. Ever since she was young, she could sense a form of tension between her inner experience, how she felt on the inside, and the biological body she was born with.

Early on, Sarah, whose given name was David, had started noticing that the clothes given to her didn't feel right on her body. "I felt like I was wearing an outfit that didn't quite fit. I could wear boys' clothes, but it didn't feel right." Sarah recalls when she was still a young boy—from a biological perspective—her dad had brought home a bag of upcycled clothing. She was very much attracted to the female clothes and dressed up in them. She had this real sense of satisfaction when putting them on.

Her dad, of a Middle Eastern culture, started taking photos for fun. But Sarah somehow felt really ashamed of these photos and didn't want to keep them. It was as if something much greater was being revealed that confused her. She wasn't quite ready to face what was going on inside her. Over many years, this brought to light a much deeper and subtler feeling of somehow being trapped in the body of the wrong gender.

As a child during Halloween, Sarah noticed how she really enjoyed dressing up as a woman. She loved playing with wigs and makeup. At first it was only for play. It came from a place of: "Hey, wouldn't it be fun to change my look?" But it brought this deep satisfaction that Sarah simply couldn't ignore. She looked at herself in the mirror and something would just release. But it was only during her makeup program in Vancouver at the age of nineteen in 2010 when it became undeniable to her.

Her teacher, who was also part of the makeup department for an international association for theatrical stage, called on Sarah to be part of a demonstration. She would direct Sarah to look straight into the mirror, and every time she did, it would sink in a little deeper—Sarah was looking straight into the eyes of a woman. Then her teacher spoke up to the class: "In terms of drag culture, you see"—she pointed to Sarah's face—"Sarah isn't too far off from looking female." This prompted Sarah to call her mom, who she talked with every night, to tell her: "You know, Mom, how you always wanted to have a girl? Now you do. That girl is me."

At first, her mom wasn't quite sure how to take this. When Sarah moved back home, her mother found her a job in the school where she worked as the vice-principal. It was at this time that

Sarah decided to start the Real Life Experience (R.L.E)—her social transition in the workplace. She started wearing makeup in public and enjoyed wearing a wig. She started buying female clothes. And as much as her mother was supportive, it was also a little disconcerting for her to have her own child begin to transition to a woman in their shared workplace.

Her mom worried that people might start talking poorly of herself and Sarah. But Sarah was full of resolve and was resilient. She consistently dressed and acted as a female. Over time, as she worked and studied in other environments, she continued as a female. For the most part, not many people seemed to mind or pay attention. Not many comments were overheard.

Another important step on her path was during a reiki session given by her cousin in 2010. This energy session was a powerful moment that opened the door to self-acceptance. Up to that point, Sarah didn't know if society or her family would accept her decision to finally come home to herself. Sarah acknowledges that it can be a really difficult thing for families to accept. When she would hear other people's stories and how they were rejected by their families, it worried her. "The reality check for me was that I was worried my family wouldn't accept me."

Sarah's parents separated when she was six. Her father had come from a small Middle Eastern village, and her mother was Catholic. Sarah eventually learned not to be burdened by her father's lectures and disapproval and just framed his views as coming from a really traditional background. He told her once, "Don't follow your heart." This comment did the opposite. It ignited Sarah's determination to follow her dream of changing genders. But Sarah didn't give up on her father for his comment.

Regardless of his lack of support, Sarah continues to reach out to him and to show understanding for his unique situation. Being a heart-centred human being, Sarah's innate capacity to understand people's pain would allow her to reach out to them with compassion. This was also true in the middle of post-op recovery with the other women at the gender reassignment recovery house. Sarah always knew when one of the girls was having a hard time, especially considering the life-altering surgery they were experiencing together, and with the tremendous stress and physical pain affecting them all.

Even as Sarah was undergoing the transformation herself, she would support someone else in need by being up for a heartfelt hug. Sarah feels like "vulnerability is a superpower," and she nails it. She is always sensitive and attentive to what is happening around her, what people are feeling and experiencing. She is continually ready to show support with a word of kindness. One of Sarah's dear friends once gave her this piece of advice: "Put love into everything you do, because that will pull you through." And this is how Sarah lives her life.

Sarah knows quite vividly what it means to pull through. "I understand why people are negative at times, but for me to survive, I have to think positively." One of the challenges that Sarah was grappling with was the fact that she didn't have many role models. "Now it has become a media sensation, but back then, I knew only a few individuals who went through with the transition," she says. She had the insecurity that comes with being a trailblazer: when the mainstream doesn't get you, you tend to second guess yourself.

At first, her family encouraged her to just enjoy cross-dressing and doing the "drag gig." But that didn't feel like it was addressing the root of the problem. It wasn't going far enough. It wasn't just about entertainment, it was this deeper need for serenity, and this meant becoming a woman. It was having a woman's body, vagina, and female hormones. This was what she desired. She also knew that her body, as it was, didn't accommodate her sexual preferences.

Sarah started hormones at the age of twenty-one with progressively cyclical levels of progesterone and estrogen in her body. "I won't have a period, but it has made my hips wider, my breasts larger and my skin softer! Everything is totally different," she says. She was finally accepted for surgery in 2018. Sarah and her mother, along with her two aunties and eldest brother, traveled to Montreal for the operation.

At the *Centre de Chirurgie de Changement de Sexe* she was greeted by a very supportive doctor. The post-op recovery took place in a convalescent home called l'Asclépiade, which means "the flower on which monarch butterflies attach themselves as they fan and unfold their wings after leaving the chrysalis."

Sarah shares that after the operation, the staff won't allow them to look at their vagina immediately. The patients must wait five days in order to let the inflammation settle down and to avoid any emotional shock. It also allows the patients to integrate all the fundamental changes that are happening to them. There is an understanding that this process is taxing on one's psychological well-being so there is a careful, step-by-step procedure to reduce overwhelming feelings. Sarah felt held and supported the whole way through and was particularly moved by the feeling of sisterhood that was experienced among patients. Everyone was going through this together. They would laugh and cry together, and extend help to each other.

As we held our interview over Skype, Sarah was resting. She still had various self-care practices that she needed to do for her gender reassignment to adequately settle in. She had various devices she needed to insert to help the newly minted vagina form properly and help it dilate as it should. Despite the physical trauma, Sarah allowed herself time to heal and adjust to her new reality. She recalls it as being a vulnerable time in her life.

Regardless of this intense experience, Sarah says, "I love my body; the transformation is extremely exciting to me. You know that you can transform your body. It feels like a futuristic thing to me. It took me years to get where I am. With this new medical knowledge and skill, it is pretty amazing that we can now allow people to align their inside and outside self. It allowed me to piece myself both physically and emotionally back together."

When I asked Sarah if she had anything else to share, she gave me this last image: "Well, you know when you've been running a marathon and you get close to the finish line, people are there on both sides of you, held behind a fence extending their hands out to you. And as you walk by them, you brush your hands against them. This is sort of what it feels like. Often you think you are alone, but really, there are always people on the sidelines rooting for you and proud of your courage."

Soul Reverb

Now that you're considering an even more fundamental view of decolonization, it's time for reflection. Reach for your workbook or journal and write down your answers.

1. Where has there been a disconnect between what people think you are and what you feel you are?
2. How has this affected how you show up for sex, and in your life? How has this inhibited you from showing up as "you"?
3. How has this affected your sense of well-being in regards to your own body and sexuality?

Chapter Affirmations

- I get to exist just as I am. I love to be my authentic self.
- When I reveal myself, I give myself permission to exist.
- When I accept who I am, others can too.
- When I give myself permission to express my authentic self, everyone benefits.

Sex Up Your Life

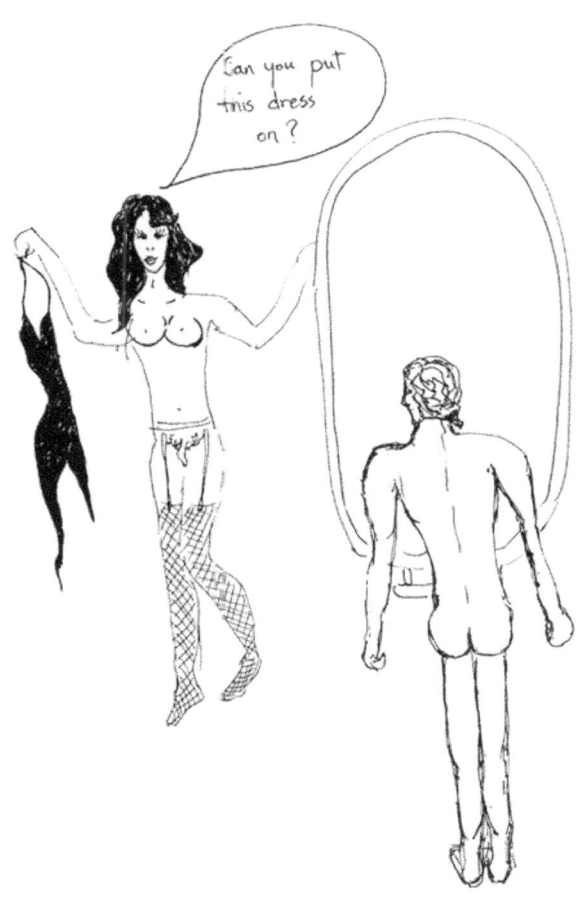

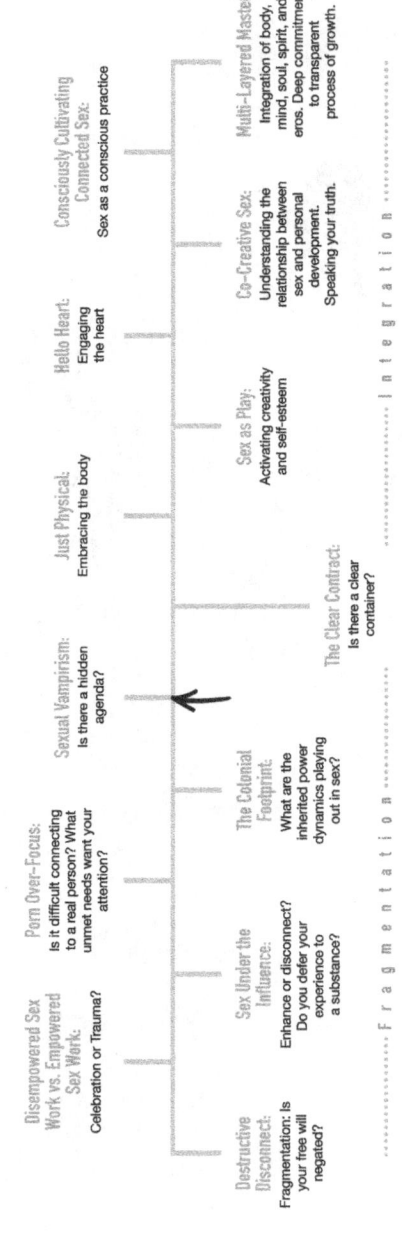

CHAPTER 6:

SEXUAL VAMPIRISM

"When you give yourself to me, completely, I will bite you. Until then, my love, I will only nibble on you."

—Tina Carreiro

To bring sex and relationships to higher levels of connection, you need to understand a very simple and yet profound principle—you need to own your shadow, which I can describe as the cloak of our insecurities. Once you've uncovered your insecurities, you need to own them and dissolve them.

If you master this, get ready for a homecoming. But the difficult thing is actually seeing your shadow, because it usually lurks in well-crafted blind spots. The shadows are created by fault lines and cracks in your being—the fragmented parts of your being. And you can bet on your shadow showing up in sex; it always does, whether you see it or not. Sex is pure energy. So whatever shadows are hiding in the recesses of your being, sex will reveal it.

Before we move onto the second half of the continuum to integrative sex, as opposed to fragmenting sex, we have one more important step: becoming conscious of our shadow and noticing how it plays out in the debilitating dynamic of Sexual Vampirism.

Sexual Vampirism

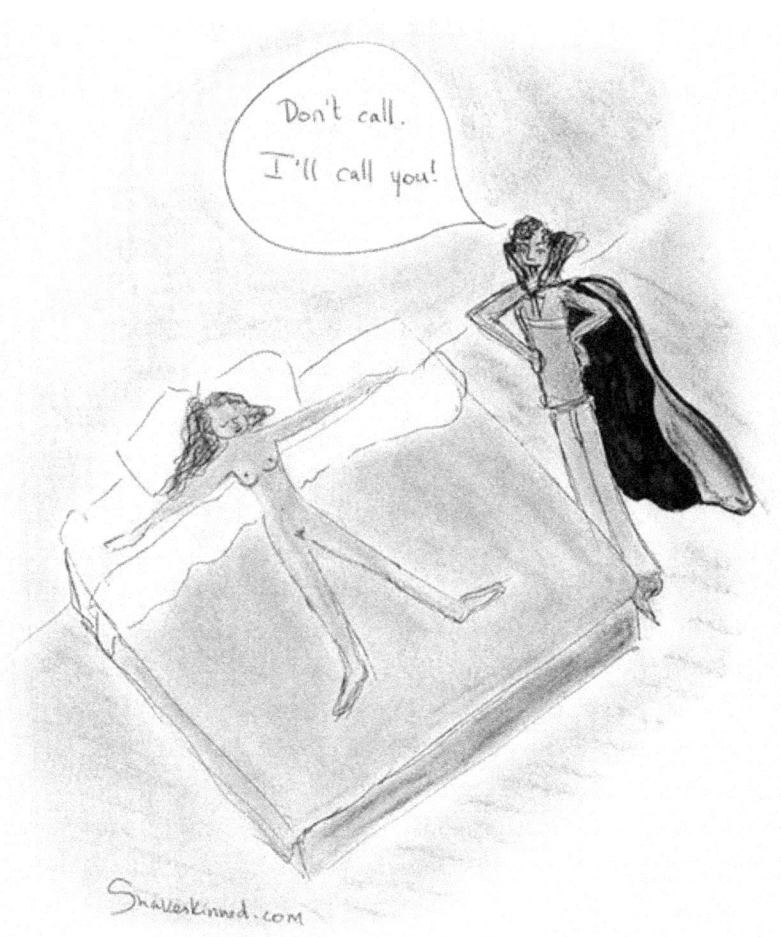

In this chapter you will:

- Learn what sexual vampirism is
- Learn how sexual vampirism happens on an energetic level
- Discover the effects of sexual vampirism and how you can begin to heal
- Experience Adriana's, Carolina's, and Marjory's stories with sexual vampirism

What is Sexual Vampirism?

Sexual Vampirism is a subtle energetic dynamic that happens much more than we are aware of. In essence, it involves sex or sexual attraction where one individual in the coupling is not disclosing their hidden intentions. To up your frequency in life, sex, and relationships, you have to get a handle on this one or else you will walk around constantly depleted. And who wants that? Not me!

This kind of sex is not straightforward physical abuse. Yet something about it is not completely straight or honest. It's sort of like discovering leeches on your body. It is not rape on the physical level, but a form of "theft" on the energetic level, which also feels like a violation once you come to see it.

It involves sex where one individual in the coupling is not disclosing their hidden intentions, as a means of getting a much-needed energy "hit." An unconscious part of the vampire's psyche is harbouring an unaddressed wound that is playing out in their behavior, a form of compensation that is unbeknownst to them. In other words, their wound is hidden in their blind spot, yet it is the driving force behind their behavior.

Sexual vampires are needy for life forces because they lack full access to their own, due to blocked energy or unresolved pain points. When you become acquainted with how energy moves in your body, you can experience the sensation of pent-up energy from unprocessed emotions and the powerful release that comes when you finally let go. This can come in the form of emotions, tears, or a simple mind shift, but the more you become aware of it, the more you become sensitive to when it happens. When I guide clients through a process, they may start our sessions with weight on their shoulders, but with addressing some of their core issues, they feel much lighter, much clearer by the end of the session. These are tangible ways of noticing how energy moves and unlocks in your body.

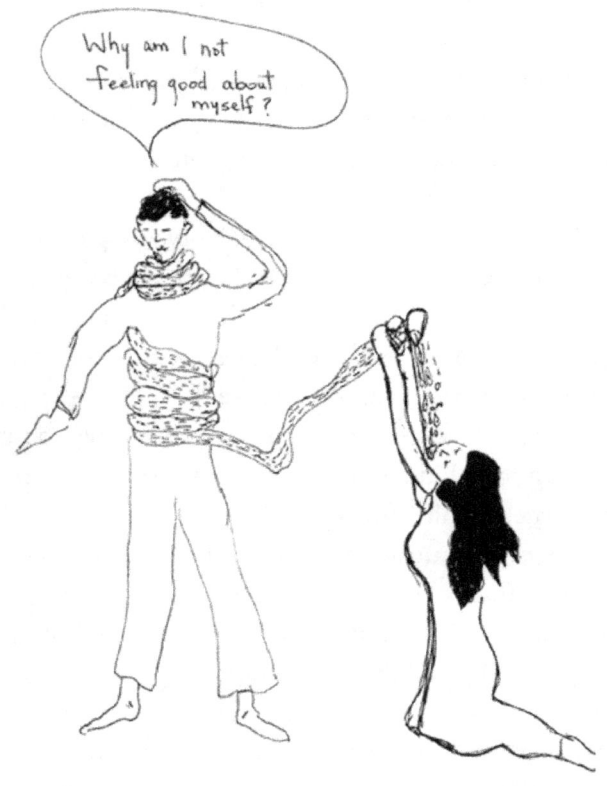

Baljit Rayat, a multi-dimensional energy healer, explained this phenomenon wonderfully on Devi Ward's radio show "Sex is Medicine." When someone is avoiding addressing emotional blockages, which ends up depleting their life forces, sex can enable them to replenish themselves by accessing someone else's life forces, or more bluntly, stealing it from them.

How do they do this? Sexual activity activates powerful life forces—chi[19]—and circulates them between two people. When one of the sexual partners is in a depleted state, they cannot contribute any energy for the exchange. Instead they are energized without actually offering any in return. They simply take. When they are satisfied, they find a way to close shop, withdraw, and leave. When they need to stock up, they return. If access is denied, they move on to someone else.

On the other hand, the person who lost the energy will experience a sudden feeling of emptiness and loss, propelling them into their own state of depletion. This sharpens their feelings of neediness and insecurity. People who have been vampirized, explains Baljit, display symptoms such as exhaustion rather than vitality. They feel anxious or hollow after sex. They might even suddenly feel emotionally needy or fears may flare up. Insecurities skyrocket while self-esteem plummets. It's the vampire, the most dominant person in the coupling, who leaves with the loot: the energy.

This energy dynamic is problematic because it can be done very smoothly without the vampirized partner noticing it at first. Sexual vampires conceal their intentions and make the other person believe, either overtly or indirectly, that they are actually loved and desired, when in fact their energy is being sapped. The sexual vampire is in a state of energetic survival. If the person was perfectly transparent and said, "I don't love you. I am just depleted

---

[19] In traditional Chinese culture, qi or ch'i is believed to be a vital force forming part of any living organism.

and too scared of taking ownership of my pain. Let me take your life forces instead so I can feel good about myself!", chances are people wouldn't go for it.

But surprisingly, some people give away their energy all the time, especially when they want to please or want to be loved… desperately. At all cost. The "vampirized" person's shadow is that they are emotionally needy. They settle for the illusion of love rather than face the truth: they crave to be loved. Most at risk are those who walk around starved for love, those who hold the belief that love is hard to find, unavailable to them, and therefore must settle. And yes, the result is costly.

Their life forces are being drained to feed someone else. The impact is that they lose the energy to move their own lives forward or to find an authentic relationship that nourishes and supports them for real. The irony of all this is that coupling with an energy vampire will leave them feeling lonelier, used, disappointed, less loved and desired than before. Since they have yielded their power to someone else, they become disempowered.

Along my journey in interviewing for this book, I came across stories like this, including extreme cases of devastation. Although I was tempted to choose the more acute stories, I decided to share examples that illustrate how common it is.

Adriana's Story—Unclear Boundaries

Adriana was a young doctor whose intense studies and commitment to her work had made it difficult for her to establish any lasting intimate relationships. She was often exhausted and overextended and had an inconsistent schedule. When she met Clive, she was quickly taken by his gusto and charm. He was a brash, opinionated artist who could generate playful humor at the flip of a coin. She was amused and impressed by his presence. But they both had deep insecurities.

For one, Adriana, not having been in a relationship for a while, worried about not being enough. Clive, while having the same worry due to a difficult previous break-up that eroded his self-esteem, exuded a bravado and confidence that blurred any traces of it. But quickly, their mutual insecurities clashed and instead of speaking about their respective worries and pains, Clive would disappear, putting Adriana in a state of panic. Her insecurities then surfaced. Was she that unlovable? Was she that unattractive? Why had he disappeared? Why wasn't he responding to her emails and text messages? Why was he avoiding her?

At first, they managed to overcome their conflicts, but as time went on, the disappearing acts multiplied. Clive would reappear after a while and they would talk about just being "friends," but their sexual connection was quite strong. And Adriana, always hopeful that they could break through their stalemates, found herself having sex with him again. But sure enough, another conflict would emerge, and the same pattern would be repeated.

When Clive came knocking on her door, she would always open it with her whole heart, hopeful that this time they could break the cycle. Weren't these eternal returns a sign of love?

Upon one return, he suggested they go jogging together and perhaps they could go for a drink afterwards. After jogging under a hot August sun, they were both drenched in sweat. The next logical step was to take a shower, which created an erotic ambiguity. Even if they were by now "officially" ex-partners, they would be naked again together under the same roof.

Adriana's sex drive was also activated by physical activity. Add a few drinks, and it sealed the deal. The sexual energy by this time was tangible and they quickly found themselves passionately entangled in sexual embrace once more. But this time, once the act was done, Clive got up and started gathering his things. Was he leaving already? This hit her in the gut. Once he left, she found herself on her bed feeling horrible. What was going on? She felt really down on herself, the voices of negativity grew, and her self-worth just plummeted. Tears ran down her face. Clive was not reachable ... again. Well, they weren't officially together, anyway, she concluded.

When she came to see me she was hemorrhaging energy, giving herself away without discernment. After a session together, she understood that when Clive would leave in such a context, it would exacerbate all her insecurities. She would feel depleted. Why was this pattern showing up in her life? As it turned out, Adriana's father had this pattern of withdrawal while she was growing up: any time issues would occur, instead of dealing with them, communicating through them, and being vulnerable, he would withdraw. He did this repeatedly with the various women in his life. Every time he started a new relationship with a woman, he was all charms and engagement. But as soon as problems would emerge, he would emotionally withdraw, often leaving little communication about why they were no longer together.

Adriana had internalized this pattern and was always hopeful for a better, more "mature" communication with men. Every time a man would withdraw from her, it put her in a state of panic and survival. To recognize this pattern in her own life was a rude awakening. She discovered that she no longer needed to play out this unconscious dynamic and run after a man who was not forthcoming and capable of authenticity. If a man was running away, it was not for her to run after him. This realization helped Adriana untie the cords that were keeping her in this unhealthy holding pattern with Clive, where she no longer needed his approval. To understand this was as if the spell had released her. She could now move on to find a relationship that would truly honor her capacity for authentic connection and communication.

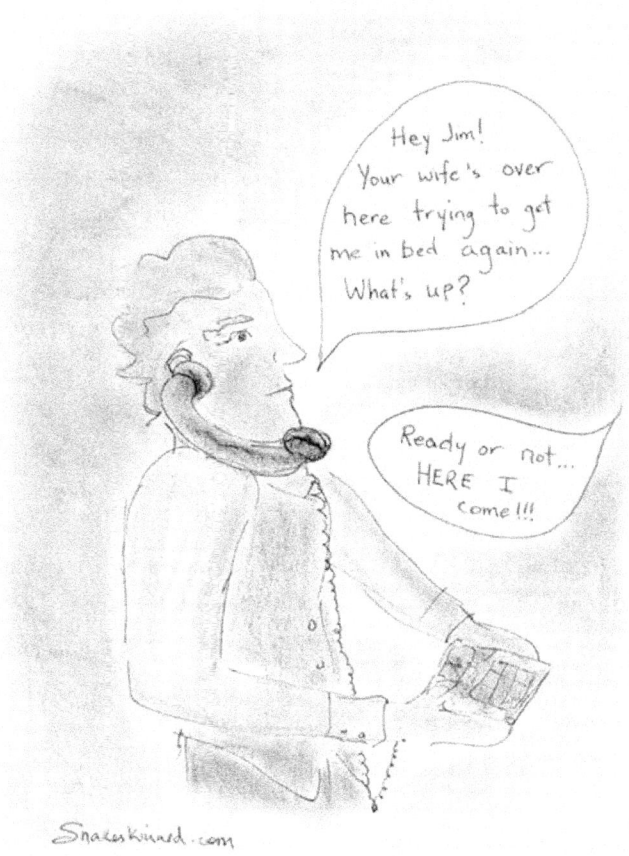

How a Vampire Hooks You In

Some of these sexual vampires may be doing this very consciously, but others may be in such a depleted state that they blindly act out of a state of energetic survival; they just know they like or want the energy. Energy gives them a boost—it's like getting a car battery jumped. But they never looked into the cause of their dead battery. Instead of fixing the cause, they would rather find another car to jump them again. And again. And again. But what if you are the car that always needs to jump that depleted battery?

These types of relationships can drag on for very long periods of time due to lack of clarity, authentic, communication, and integrity. The vampire's strategy is to keep the relationship in a gray zone, which makes maneuvering that much easier.

This is exactly what happens in cheating relationships. The cheater, not addressing whatever true concerns exist in their committed relationship, finds a new secret liaison to fulfill some unaddressed void. They then feed all kinds of illusions to the new lover, keeping them hooked in the dynamic without ever taking action on the initial problems in their committed relationship. Nor do they typically take steps to end it. "I love you, but I can't leave my partner ... just yet!" Sound familiar? This is the definition of ambiguity; continuing to engage but with a lack of clarity while activating juicy stashes of sexual energy. The end result is most often the same: emotional depletion and exposure to long periods of energy loss.

This is where cheating and the principles of polyamory differ. In polyamory, the lovers agree to create a container for themselves and the other lovers involved. They establish, in principle, transparent agreements in an ethical way. If you have an agreement, and follow through on it, you are protecting the relationships from energetic theft and leakage. You may need to readjust and communicate along the way to accommodate new needs as they emerge. In this way, the container remains solid for all involved. With a clear, open agreement, you ensure that everyone feels safe, and that the energetic transactions are transparent. This way, betrayal can be avoided.

Carolina's Story—Cheating

Sexual vampirism can be very subtle; so camouflaged that we usually don't see it when it's happening. Carolina fell head over heels for a subtle and suave man. He had rented a room in her flat while he was on a business trip for his Silicon Valley high-tech company. Chris was smart, handsome, and stylish. But most of all, he seemed to know how to connect with her. As it turned out, he was somewhat of an empath, meaning someone who is highly attuned to people's emotions and experiences. They were both introverted, and it was blissful for Carolina to find someone else with such a compatible inner world. The only problem was that he was in a long-term committed relationship.

Regardless, Chris seemed to really enjoy Carolina's company, and she was single and missing intimate touch. As it turned out, Chris was very much needing it too. Apparently, his partner didn't like to cuddle, and he longed for that. One night, as they talked, he lay on his belly, stretched out on the ground. Carolina could feel the energetic pull. He wanted her to touch him. She resisted at first, but the attraction grew between them. He invited her to join him for meals at local trendy restaurants. Then he gave her a ticket to join him at a rock concert. The romance of fine dining and concerts just amplified their connection. The joys seemed endless and the emotional intimacy multiplied exponentially. And finally, a simple massage turned into a series of deep, loving cuddles and kisses.

When he returned home, he would re-work his schedule to secretly spend hours talking over Skype with Carolina. He told her he had fallen in love and that he had to come back and spend time with her to find out if they should be together, but he couldn't tell his partner the real motive of his travels. Enamored, Carolina went for it. They seemed to connect so deeply. She believed he may indeed be the man she had been waiting for. Everything seemed so perfect, minus a clear relationship status.

But when he returned, different things started to feel off. One night, instead of feeling replenished by his cuddles, she woke up feeling like she was going to literally suffocate in his embrace. His arms were wrapped around her, and all she could think of doing was removing herself from what felt like an energy vacuum. How could this be possible with someone who she was so fond of? This almost made her second guess herself and the sensations she was having. But she could not ignore it; if she did not move out of that energy vortex, and fast, it felt like she would literally wither and die.

Of course, Chris was deeply offended and accused her of not liking to cuddle; how could they possibly foresee a future together? Carolina, who wanted to please him, was dumbfounded. Little did she know that this behavior was called 'gaslighting,' a form of manipulation, discrediting her experiences with nonsensical accusations. Instead of owning his own fears, which were well activated from his primary relationship, he would make Carolina feel like she was wrong for moving away from him and tending to her needs.

It was also a form of undercover threat: *if you need to pull away from me, you are not a good fit for me*. He was projecting onto her all his own insecurities. The truth was that he was feeling depleted and rejected by his primary partner, so instead of trying to understand his issue and addressing his feelings of emasculation by his partner, he was trying to feed off a new woman to regain his sense of worth. It was also a great set-up for triangulation: creating a dynamic to play one against the other.

When she came for a consult, she understood that Chris had his own issues to take care of. For one thing, he was in a relationship where his partner dominated him, which triggered some of his unresolved mother issues. His mother, unhappy in her marriage, would turn to him, as he was a sensitive boy, and almost feed off his energy. He needed to push her away. The interesting thing was that in his relationship to his primary partner, she was the one pushing him away. And when she wouldn't give him what he wanted, he turned to Carolina, who seemed at first to be giving and generous.

Carolina also had her share of responsibility in this affair. She went for the bait. She was needy as well and had wounds that blinded her from the initial signs. Her own childhood family dynamics led her to falsely believe that perhaps no one would ever be attracted to her or love her. So when this handsome and smart man came along and they were hitting it off like two soulmates, she fell for the illusion. But one thing was clear; her body knew it all along. One night, just as her delusion was starting to fade, she found herself crouched over the toilet bowl throwing up. She had been used, not loved.

Boundaries

When you no longer want to tolerate the ambiguity implicit in sexual vampirism and want out, you will attempt to establish new boundaries or withdraw. At this time, the vampire will most likely extend another hook, another temptation to reignite your hope. *Hey! Don't leave, you are special to me...* But if you bite again, which you may (it happens all the time), you will also notice that nothing of the ambiguous state has actually changed. The energy vampire is after the life forces and the feeling they provide them, not you as a person!

The interesting thing is that when you stop deferring your power to the un-transparent partner and stop your energetic leakage, they may actually be angry with you as you are taking away their stash of tasty and comforting life forces. But again, don't confuse this with love. They were relying on you for their survival, as an addict would a drug. They really need their fix, after all. They will seek out someone else willing to stoke their energy fire for them. The good news is if you manage to sever your codependence, your energy will come back to you with self-care. Your confidence will climb if you look into your own unconscious pain to stop attracting energy vampires. When you uncover your own shadow, you will heal.

Let's look into another form of sexual vampirism, when sexual energy is used to extort or covertly get something from someone else.

Marjory's Story—Love Fraud

Marjory came in for a consultation regarding some odd sexual experiences. She hadn't had a sexual relationship for over twenty-five years. And yet, out of the blue, she started waking up in the middle of the night and feeling like a presence was having sex with her. It literally felt like something was stroking her clitoris. She had been on a journey to heal her sexuality and needed some clarity about it all.

One of the first things that became clear in our session was that Marjory was very open but was unaware of how her energy was dissipating. She was a highly spiritual person, and yet her intuition, her trust in herself and in what she was experiencing, were eroded. She found herself in relationships that would "use her" while not clueing in that it would be better for her to leave them before they seriously damaged her—financially.

She had married a man who had trouble being responsible for his life. He let her get the corporate job, at which she excelled. He justified staying home for the kids, but she quickly found out that it was his way of opting out of responsibilities and indulging in pot smoking. Over time, he grew increasingly belligerent and angry. She grew more depressed and powerless to change anything as she became energetically drained. After years of not having sex with her, he decided to file for a divorce. She had become quite fearful of what he would do and decided to simply sign the divorce papers, which said she would not get any child support in exchange for not losing half her retirement fund.

After the divorce, she met another man. He quickly lured her with charm, his sexual energy and spiritual discourse, and when she was on his hook, he asked her for a loan for his ailing business. It started off as a small amount but added up to $75,000 in total. When it was time to reimburse Marjory, he hired a lawyer and filed a lawsuit against her for usury, which he managed to win. Not only did he win the case, but she would have to pay him another $75,000. Marjory filed for bankruptcy.

I share this story simply to illustrate what happens when your energy is drained by an energy vampire. Obviously these two men knew they could get what they needed without taking responsibility for their own lives. Rather, they not only made Marjory work for it, but pay for it too. And although Marjory was discontent with what was happening, she remained in the relationships until the men decided to leave her.

In both cases, she discharged her energy to them, made quite visible by the large sums of money she gave them with no returns. Here the sexual vampirism takes on a different nuance, that of love fraud. Sex is used to initiate an intimate relationship with the sole purpose of usurping her. Sex and sexual energy here are used to seal the deal.

Marjory's self-esteem and sense of well-being crashed. In our session, it became clear that growing up with an alcoholic father had warped her sense of boundaries. She was acting as the little girl who looked up to Daddy with loving eyes, seeing his pain and wanting to do something for him. It was growing up wanting to be extra good for her father's affection and love, and always hoping that he would change. The problem was, this "good little girl" was letting energy vampires eat her up.

When she finally grasped her error, she was shaken. "I just cannot get over that something I thought was a positive is actually a negative ... the good girl," she wrote to me after our session. Indeed. This is the surprising power of releasing the belief systems that don't serve us. What we were taught to think was good can be the very belief system that is hurting us.

While the examples I collected have mostly been from women's points of view, anyone can be an energy vampire. It isn't a gendered phenomenon. Many men have shared feeling used by women sexually in all kinds of scenarios.

A Thai friend of mine shared, for example, that she knew of women courting more than one international men at a time while not being upfront about it. They owned several cell phones to maintain the illusion that they were "committed" to them to financially gain from as many sources as possible. Here we have the traditional 'gold digger' idea where "a person dates others purely to extract money from them, in particular a woman who strives to marry a wealthy man"[20]. In this scenario, women prey on vulnerable or lonely men for their financial gain.

Anytime there is manipulation, inauthenticity, taking advantage of someone to get something, whether it be money, prestige, or energy hit, combined with activated sexual energy, you're lining up for sexual and energetic vampirism. Sexual vampirism exists where there are hidden agendas running the show. It can be as simple as the energy vampire seeking sexual validation because they do not feel good about themselves or they lack self-worth.

But let's also recall who took the bait and why: the "energy leaker" is needy to be loved. Seeing the whole picture allows you to break the spell.

---

20 https://www.lexico.com/en/definition/gold_digger

How to Apply This to Your Life

The good news is that you are only an energy vampire when you don't want to deal with what is hidden underneath. If you get to the root problem, if you finally take responsibility for your own pain and heal it, rather than projecting it on others or suppressing it or opting for the crutch, i.e. stealing it from someone else, your energy fills back up. You are no longer in a deficit mode, but fully replenished, grounded in yourself and ready to engage healthily with others.

Understanding this is key to improving the quality of your sexual experiences and life. It also reveals another fundamental truth—our sex lives and our personal development are intimately connected. To leave the realm of disempowered or fragmenting sex, one needs to enter the zone of clarity, lucidity, and self-respect.

When Issues Fester

Sexual Vampirism is comparable to being in an addictive state, and if not tended to, can get pretty devastating. Eva Pierrakos explains in her book *Creating Union* that someone with really deep-set energy blocks can experience forms of sexual deviance. These types of energy vampires may strike even more vulnerable groups, including children. We all know that children have remarkable energy—fresh and lively—that allow them to grow. When sexual predators turn to children to plunder their energy, the results can be extremely disturbing and harmful to the children involved.

Those who grow up with sexual abuse in their childhood often lose their vivaciousness and energy and have to restore it through coaching or therapy. They feel that their sex/vitality/energy/creativity is dangerous, so they become depressed when really expressing self is what saves them. It is not uncommon for survivors to become perpetrators if unaddressed.

The reality is that there are many depleted people roaming this earth for sex who don't know how to take responsibility for themselves. But there are just as many people leaking their energy and hoping to be loved from such illusions. They too need to own their shadow. They too are needy and depleted. One attracts the other. It is not surprising that vampire movies like the Twilight saga make a killing in the box office. This series alone grossed $3.3 billion in worldwide receipts! If you look more closely, you will notice that this play between the energy vampire and the energy leaker explains a large percentage of sexual behavior in the world.

Sex on "Family" Duty

There is one other permutation of sexual vampirism that I want to explore. It is an even subtler energetic dynamic, since it happens within the confines of an established, perhaps legally bound, desired relationship. No malicious wrongdoing occurs, but rather lack of consciousness and proper boundaries. I will call this dynamic "Sex on Duty." A few clients of mine have brought this to the table. They are in a relationship they want, they love their partner, and yet, over time they become seriously depleted: depressed, anxious, and with a loss of sexual desire.

Often they have had children, are most likely the primary caregiver at home, and are drained by the relentless and never-ending job of childrearing and home-keeping. They don't have a fulfilling job outside the home, which would get them out of the house, and exchanging with other adults, so there is an element of isolation. This occupation also has responsibilities that can often remain somewhat invisible.

Now, let's put sex into the picture. Their partner comes home from a long day at work, and as the lights go out, would love some sexual relief from their stresses. The primary caregiver and household keeper, in the role of constantly giving, also believes she must tend to her partner's needs, and yet the last thing on earth she wants is sex. She is simply exhausted from her day.

But believing it is her duty to please her partner and satisfy him sexually, she lets it happen. She isn't fully into it, and yet she yields to his desires and hides her lack of interest because she is on duty, albeit quite clearly on overtime. She just cooperates with his desires, his wants. What a few clients have noted is that over time, this wears them out. They talk to me about "needing to satisfy their husband's needs 'just because' he has needs."

The "Exhausted Mom"

"If young moms don't have enough support, I think our brains are wired to be in survival mode, well-domesticated survival mode, with constant thoughts about all the things you could have forgotten or done wrong during the day. The constant insecurity keeps you drained. Babies and children sense this. Therefore, they often respond to their mom's insecurities by being even more needy or clingy. And some moms take this as a sort of comfort and even put their child between them and their partner. I have seen this twice with mom-son relationships—really uncomfortable to be around. But back to the lack of sex. I remember many nights where I just rolled over to 'get it done' because I felt guilty not initiating sex when my child was young. The worst part was that I never confided in anyone because I presumed this was how it was supposed to be." These were her "wifely duties", an idea that can be traced back to religious dogmas and cultural traditions.

So here is the deal. Sex is a heightened exchange of life forces. When you are depleted from all your day's activities, from lack of fulfillment, from lack of support, from insecurities, your life force barometer is at LOW. And did you know that children also feed off your energy stash to build their own? In this case, it's a healthy growing mechanism, which also demands a healthy self-care

Sexual Vampirism

practice to replenish. This is at its highest peak between the ages of birth and age six. No wonder you are exhausted, right? Now, add in "giving" sex because you think it is your duty.

You are "giving" again when the tank is already close to empty. If you are entering a sexual exchange that is not a mutual experience, or mutually desired; you are just going to leak what you've got, and it might even put you in deficit mode. One partner takes, the other one gives up. There is a transfer of energy from the duty-bound one to the one initiating, which won't be helpful in the long run. Since the duty-bound partner is already depleted, it may, over time, tip them into depression or unhealthy habits. It may mean they start drinking alcohol to get some relief. They may start compensating to get a hit of energy from someone else.

And if your truth is compromised, whereby you don't tell your partner what is really going on, the connection is not happening in the relationship either and connection will be eroded. Your feeling of duty may eventually ruin the sexual current that once beautifully bound you together. And when that happens, it may lead to other unfortunate situations. Cheating is one of them. A healing crisis is another possibility. And just think about it—how can someone be attracted to you if you are super depleted? All your juiciness is gone.

So, the energetic vampirism here happens because sex is playing out in a very unconscious way. To remedy this situation requires maturity. It requires re-evaluating all the energetic dynamics and transactions happening throughout the day to address where the leaks are happening. First and foremost, this demands honest and open communication of needs. It could be as simple as finding activities that allow them both to replete their energy stashes, such as some physical activity, a walk in nature. It could even be meditation. There is more on that in the chapter on cultivating a conscious practice. The bottom line is that it requires a lot of honesty and realism.

Self-care needs to be a priority here. The goal: to nurture and nourish your life forces. Let them grow. Let them overflow. Then, share and enhance them. Sex, when it is coming from a place of fullness and of shared desire, multiplies life forces exponentially. Ultimately, when you start noticing that you are becoming depleted, this is an invitation to deepen and learn what is happening. You will be surprised what you discover!

Soul Reverb

Now that you're seeing sexual vampirism in action and are aware of its effects and what is needed for healing, it's time for reflection. Reach for your workbook or journal and write down your answers.

1. Have you ever had an energy vampire take your energy? Did you notice how it made you feel?
2. Do you know why you were leaking your energy?
3. What state is your intuition in? Do you override its messages? What's your payoff to staying blind?

If you have identified yourself as the energy vampire, consider these:

1. Have you ever manipulated someone to have sex because you needed to "get" energy or feel good about yourself?
2. Do you know why you are energetically depleted?
3. What issues are you avoiding looking at? What are you avoiding taking care of?

Chapter Affirmations

- Energy leaker: I am fully responsible for my leaky pipes.
- Energy vampire: I am fully responsible for my state of depletion.

- Energy leaker: I deserve a relationship with someone who can take ownership of their fears and insecurities, as opposed to projecting them on me, and sucking me dry.
- Energy vampire: I need to own my pain and take care of it. I am fully responsible for myself.
- Both: If I am feeling scared or insecure, I get to find the root cause and self-soothe or ask for support.

The Lower Continuum: When Sex Fragments Us

We've unpacked a lot of the unconscious dynamics playing out in sex. Do any of these dynamics show up in your life? Start noticing what part of you gets fragmented when you have sex: Where does your body shut down, your self-esteem muddied, your natural playfulness inhibited, your heart trampled? Notice where shame wedges itself in your sexuality, where "free will" is taken or given away. Start flagging those energy leaks! When you fully appreciate the reality of what is going on, sex can leave the domain of fragmentation and enter that of integration, which is similar to putting the pieces of a puzzle back together.

Once you fully embrace the broken vase on the ground, you can start bringing the pieces back together.

Sexual energy in the absence of free will leads to destruction, whereas when it is aligned to it, this unleashes tremendous healing power.

PART 2.

SEX ON THE UPPER CONTINUUM

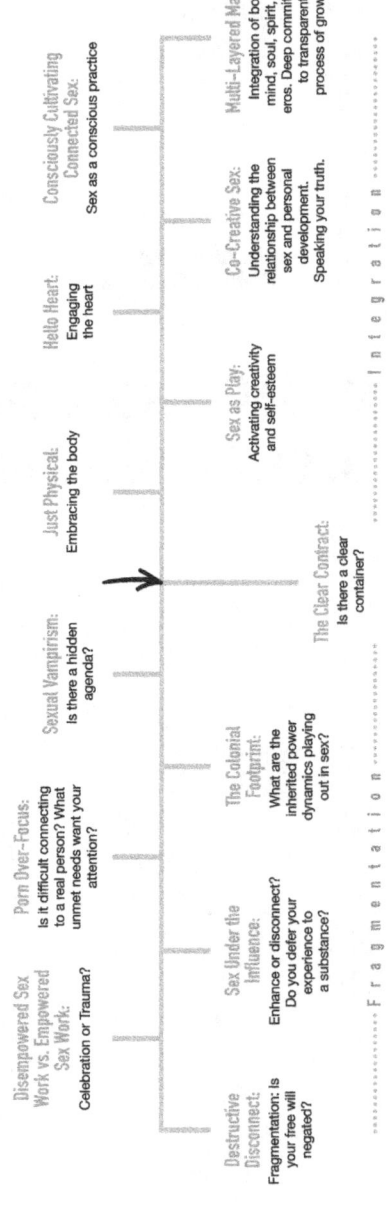

THE CLEAR CONTAINER

"Love yourself enough to set boundaries. Your time and energy are precious. You get to choose how you use it. You teach people how to treat you by deciding what you will and won't accept."

— Anna Taylor

Let's go back to that picture of the broken vase we looked at when we started. Pieces are scattered. Depending on what you've experienced in your life, this may be a good snapshot of your state. You may not even be fully aware of it. All you know is that you aren't feeling that great, your life is not where you want it to be, and the relationships and sex in your life are not fulfilling or supportive.

Let's look at the world of ancient Egyptian mythology to find our way onto the next part of the Continuum of Connection. Here, sex becomes a powerful ally to growth, to rebuilding the integrity of your entire being, your vase, and container of life.

The Egyptian myth of Isis and Osiris will illustrate what needs to happen to inch or leap across from the Lower to the Upper Continuum. It will help us understand what is involved in reassembling the shattered vase.

The Clear Container

Osiris was a good king and commanded the respect of everyone on Earth. But Set was deeply envious and jealous of his brother Osiris, because Set did not command the same innate respect. He envied Osiris for his wisdom while despising him for his goodness. Osiris was a thorn in Set's existence, so he decided to take on a human form to destroy him. He devised a plan to usurp his brother's throne. To carry out his plan, Set secretly had a wooden chest built to Osiris's measurements. Then he sent a message to Osiris saying: "Are we not brothers? Let us live in peace and friendship from here on. Let us have a banquet to celebrate our new friendship."

Osiris accepted and Set arrived at the banquet with seventy-two of his warriors. After much revelry, Set revealed his marvelous chest carved in wood and adorned with gold. He invited all attendees to see if the tomb might fit them. Of course, it fit none but Osiris. Set turned to his brother and asked him to give it a try. The coffin was a perfect fit. When Osiris lay down, Set quickly closed the coffin on his brother and his warriors nailed it closed. Set cruelly ordered that his brother's body be cut to pieces and scattered across the Nile River.

Take note: Fragmentation

But little did Set realize how deep Queen Isis's love was for her husband. She was determined to find every remnant of Osiris' body. She combed the river and collected every piece of his body found intertwined in the reeds along the river. Between rocks. Stranded on the yellow sand. She did not leave one stone unturned. She managed to gather all the pieces back together—minus the phallus—and by the power of her love for him, mended him back to life.

Take note: Integration.

And Osiris's surprising glue? Her love and intent.

With this powerful tale, we are entering new and exciting territory: Sex on the Upper Continuum! We are leaving the unconscious shadow that fragments us into pieces, behind, and gearing up to achieve blissful, authentic connection. The next chapters recount stories of sexual integration where alienated pieces of ourselves are welcomed back into their rightful place and empower us in retrieving a more complete experience of who we are.

We are sexual, physical, emotional, soulful, and spiritual beings.

To be whole, we need free will, a thriving body and sexuality, unleashed creative forces, power and confidence, a pulsating heart, and a courageous voice. We need to trust our intuition and higher perceptions. Our potential is so much greater than what we are accustomed to believing. When all these elements start working together as a whole, we access profound experiences both sexually and in our everyday lives.

First, we must establish a safe and clear container; in other words, agree to the type of energy exchange we want. The strength of our communication and respect of boundaries determine the quality of the container, hence the sexual contract.

How do we establish a container that is clear and authentic? As in any exchange, agreements can be as simple as deciding on the nature of the sexual exchange. We could agree to have physical sex, nothing more—the raw and fast booty call. But as our desires grow, we may want to increase our pleasure with playfulness and creativity. We may involve our power, invest our sense of self-worth, and confidence into building something deeper. We may notice a tingle in our heart at some point. As the experience of sex broadens, the invitation is to speak the truth of what we want and don't want clearly.

As we work up the Sex Continuum, the shadow doesn't disappear, but here there is a courageous commitment to transparency. Knowing what the "deal" involves allows people to choose what works for them. When we hide our true intentions, we slip back into sexual vampirism.

The Clear Container

Clear agreements include any kind of sexual activity, whether it be within a monogamous or polyamorous framework, under any guise: kink, BDSM, play parties, bathhouse sex, flings, sex in exclusive committed relationships, sex in wedlock, or in open marriages. As long as the agreements and protocols are clear for the consenting people, sex thrives on the Upper Continuum as a force of integration.

Often, as the relationships unfold and take form, the agreements need revision. As new needs surface, unimagined emotions wake up, unforeseen dynamics appear, clear agreements are required to adjust and be re-negotiated. Relationships are fluid and alive! And we all know that disagreements emerge. Here, on the Upper Continuum, we know this is part of the process.

The more we involve ourselves, the higher the likelihood of touching some of those dormant land mines buried inside us—the unattended wounds. Sex can and will wake up the wounding. Sex is pure energy, after all, being blasted through our bodies. Hurtful words, powerful emotions, disappointments, and fear leave an imprint in the body. When we care for the surfacing hurt, we are on the rewarding path of integration. The higher the stakes, the higher returns.

Soul Reverb

With this in mind, reach for your workbook or journal and jot down your answers.

1. At what level of your being do you truly want to engage in sexual connection? Do you recognize your soul's needs at this point in time? What are they?
2. What would a clear container look like for you right now? What do you need to communicate to your partner before diving into your next sexual experience to honor your truth?

3. If you tune into yourself, what is holding you back from having a satisfying sex life, relationship, and partnerships? What stops you from having a powerful life?

Affirmations:

- When I create clear containers for my sexual expression, I am free to receive pleasure, love, and respect.
- I am present in every moment of this experience.
- I enter into clear, mutually respectful connections with grace and ease.

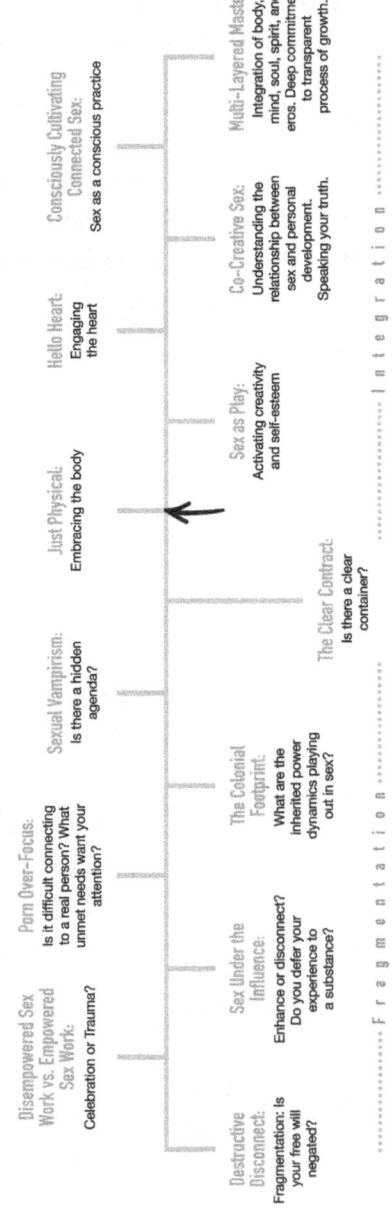

CHAPTER 7:

INHABIT YOUR BODY

"Man wanted a home, a place for warmth, or comfort, first of physical warmth, then the warmth of the affections."
—Henry David Thoreau, *Walden*

Physical sex is merely the mechanics of sex, without the involvement of the other parts of your being—no heart, no feelings, no spiritual connection, just the bare basics of rubbing each other's genitals and having a sexual release. It's the stripped-down act of copulation. Here you simply need a consenting body to channel your erotic bodily experience. We have left the sphere of sexual vampirism in being intentional and explicit about our agreement.

In this chapter you will:

- Experience Sacha's story with physical sex
- Explore the importance of embodiment
- Understand the power of permission

With physical sex, sexual partners have agreed that they do not want anything else but physical sex; the goal is not to deepen or enrich a relationship with sex, but rather the point of contact is simply the act itself, the rest is unwanted. They have agreed to get aroused by each other's bodies and its erotics. They only want to experience that fleeting moment of sexual and physical intensity. The act of sexual engagement is separated from any real relationship, or from cultivating love.

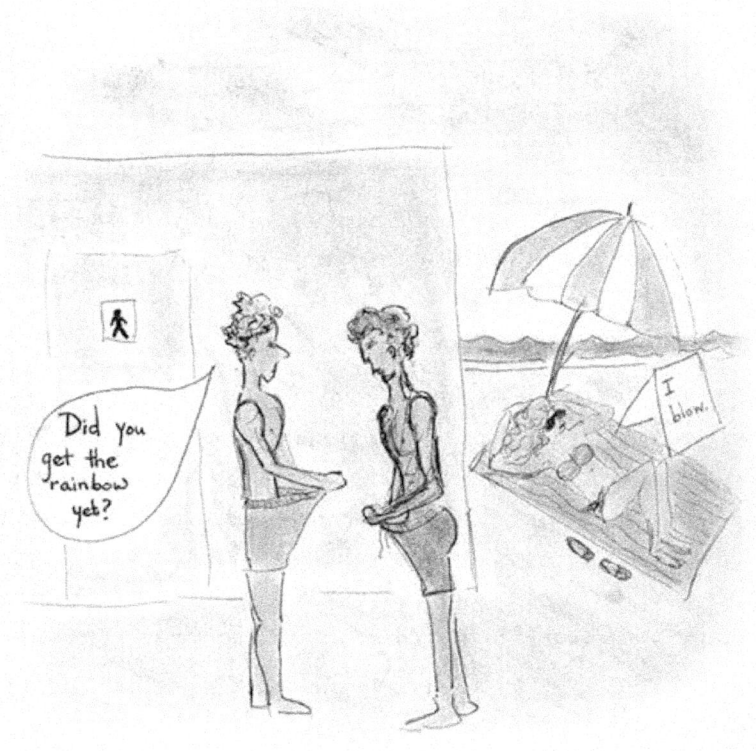

Yet, as humans with emotions, a soul life and spirit, it is hard to remain in this situation for long, if at all. We naturally seek integration of our whole being—unless completely blocked off from our feelings, or if trauma is so great we have simply disconnected from our inner selves.

At this degree of intimacy, we are simply allowing our body to have a sexual experience. We let our body feel pleasure. For many, the simple act of "feeling" pleasure in the body is a huge hurdle to overcome. Feeling good and sexual in your own body, allowing your sexual self to be expressed, embraced, and embodied is in itself healing. How can we have sex if we are not willing to share our body and let it have a sexual, erotic experience? Just think of the number of people who have shut down their sexuality once and for all! The *Washington Post* reports that 28% of men and 18% of women between the ages of 18-30 are not having sex.

The body is the interface for sex whether at its most basic level or highest forms of sexual exchange. Many cultural and religious dogmas have tried to de-sexualize the human body, basically condemning sexual pleasure as a legitimate practice, suggesting that the body was conceived simply for its biological function of procreation. When in fact, erotic pleasure is everybody's birthright. Pleasure is a portal to higher states which we will address in subsequent chapters.

Many sex educators and sex-positive activists around the world want to expand safe spaces for bodies to express sexuality by removing stigma and shame. They are creating situations where people are given the permission to explore the erotic pleasures of their body and permission to truly experience sexual pleasure.

For example, one episode of Zoë Ligon's show "Sex Stuff" illustrated techniques of Japanese bondage. If we remove the context around bondage, and simply consider it as a physical experience, being tied up gives you a bodily sensation. You can explore erotic feelings that emerge from having your body roped up, constricted. This is a simple example of discovering the erotics of your body. As much as this may be a disconcerting thought for many, if done within the context of consent—stripping it of any power dynamics—it is simply a bodily sensation, and this constriction will be pleasurable for some.

In exploring sex as a merely physical experience, powerful sexual energy is activated. As the thrust of energy is driven through the body, it may bolster feelings related to the body such as how you value it or how it's been treated in the past. It can reveal how willing you are to receive pleasure, to relax into your body's experience, how much it can surrender to pleasure or how much it is run by fear. It can reveal your capacity to mindfully tune into your body or if you tune out and disconnect from it. The physicality of sex can show how present you are in your body or if you are in a constant state of distraction. As these dynamics surface, they present the opportunity to further understand your relationship to your body and where more care, attention, and healing may be needed. Instead of disassociating, here you are embodying.

Flipping Body Shame

What about body shame? We know that body shame is a very real consideration for many people before having sex, and a real experience during sex. "Will he think I'm fat?" "Will she think my penis is too small?" These considerations can literally inhibit people from sharing themselves with others. This is why I was so fascinated with my partner's good friend who was a larger woman seemingly with no problem whatsoever in landing handsome men for sex. In fact, my partner always jokes: "I don't know how she does it, but she gets more ass than a toilet seat!" All this attention amuses and delights her. Wanting to get to the bottom of this, I asked her: "Have you ever experienced body shame?"

"Yes, she said, and I still deal with it at times, but I realized that it only takes a simple mind shift, a flip of a dime, and I can get out of thinking that way. You see, our bodies are really well designed, they are designed for pleasure, and I know that." She chuckles. "The guys that come with me discover that pretty quick too!" She laughs again. What I get from this is that she is a master at giving herself permission, and this makes her incredibly magnetic. Men from across the continent all want a piece of her. Laughing, she shares her dance card. It's quite the line up.

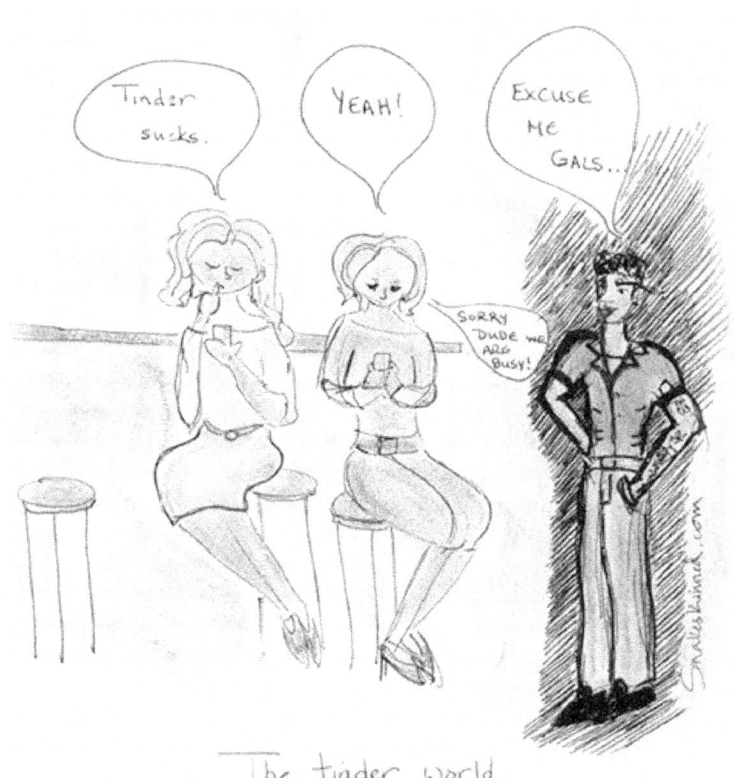

The tinder world.

What's Going on for You?

Does your sexual energy carry a lot of negative associations? Is it loaded with shame, or does it welcome fun and pleasure? You may become more aware of your body's needs, desires, and responses. This is all valuable information for your process of integration.

Shame can really drain the natural vitality of your sexual energy and can impede your natural body experience. Any traces of fight, freeze, or flight will shut down your body's sexual experience. But this isn't necessarily something to avoid! Where there is inhibition, there is useful information for you.

Your body is your home. These experiences allow you to start sensing to what degree you are at home in your own body and what is needed to support its integration.

Hidden Needs

When wanting "physical sex," unconsciously the psyche may be attempting to meet other needs. I've heard people say that they just want "sex" but then have a sense of disappointment because they are not fully satiated. They were ultimately craving other needs that were more deeply hidden: a deeper relationship, deeper intimacy, perhaps even love, but they simply do not know how to go there. In many ways, it's easier to settle for the accessibility of physical sex. This is frequently accompanied by doubt about worthiness or the right to desire more fulfilling experiences. Perhaps, the choice to engage in such an arrangement is secretly accompanied by the hope that the encounter may ultimately lead to more.

The reality of this type of arrangement lies in the disposable factor: sex merely for sex, having a physical experience, with no desire for any connection on the soul level. If you fail to set clear intentions here, you will most likely sink into the murky and depleting grounds of sexual vampirism.

You must stay conscious of what is happening for you. With physical sex your body may be getting a workout, a climax, and that is what satisfies you in that moment. But pay attention to your experience afterwards as well. By neglecting all the other parts of your being, you may ultimately feel hollow. Over time, you may want to engage your playfulness, your self-esteem, and perhaps even your heart. If you are feeling this, it has most likely awakened your desire to expand towards more involved levels of connection.

On the other hand, physical sex may be just what is needed in this precise moment of your life. This was the case for Sacha.

Sacha's Story—Embodying Pleasure

Sacha had gotten back into the dating game after a painful erosion of her long-term relationship—that led to having a child—resulting in discord and accusations.

Sacha started going on a few dates with a new man she met through Tinder with the intent of simply satisfying her sexual drive. She didn't want anything serious. As she started sleeping with Mark, she grew to realize she liked him very much and her feelings grew more intense. She decided to reveal this sentiment to Mark and apparently, he was fine with this. But as time went by, she experienced hot and cold behavior from him. Sometimes, he seemed to be withdrawing from her, which would put her in a state of panic. A voice in her head would ask: "What is wrong with me?" "Why do men always withdraw from me?"

Eventually, the hot-cold dance became unbearable for Sacha and they decided to simply be friends. But then, when they spent time together, she would end up sleeping with him again. Sacha grew irritated with herself. After she slept with him, she clearly didn't feel good. She decided to sever the "friendship" because she knew she couldn't resist having sex with him and it was not serving her. Mark put up a fight. He started calling her and acting quite nice again.

Sacha's agitation came from her fear of being tormented again. What if he withdrew from her again? It seemed impossible for her to be friends with him without slipping. She also berated herself for shutting out the friendship. Was she being mean and inflexible? Was she blocking a genuine possibility?

In our consultation, we saw how difficult it was for her to establish clear boundaries, which brings us back to the unclarity present in sexual vampirism. She had the tendency of over giving, then angrily pushing men away because she felt rejected. When her fears became her reality, she would then compensate by setting up walls as a way of protecting herself.

As we deepened her insights, her relationship with her father became a focus. When she reached puberty, her father had withdrawn from her and had become depressed. It was as if she had become invisible to him. The pain came from the fact that her body was changing. She was becoming a woman and needed to be acknowledged and accepted by her father, but he wasn't capable of doing this for her. Furthermore, her family made dating a boy seem like a shameful thing.

Once when she had been on the phone with a boyfriend her mother interrupted and told her to hang up immediately. Sacha had learned that her sexual energy was somehow shameful, and if she wanted to experience boys, she would have to do it secretly. As a teen, Sacha shared that a therapist had encouraged her to go and unburden her heart with her father by telling him how angry she was with him.

But when she did, he listened in a distant way and told her that nothing would change, and that was that. All her fire, her passion, her sexual energy, was crying to be seen, acknowledged, and valued, but every attempt she made was met with a closed door, or worse, lack of interest. She enveloped herself in a profound feeling of invisibility. From that point on, part of her being went into hiding because she believed something must be wrong with her.

In our session, I suggested she imagine talking to her father as if he were there. Tears choked her up, yet she pushed through and started asking the following questions: "Why don't you like me? Why do you ignore me? Why do you shut me out? Tell me, what's wrong with me?" These questions would come up all the time whenever she was in a relationship with a man.

She came to realize that after such a difficult break-up, she actually didn't want to get back into another significant relationship just yet. All she wanted to do was enjoy sex with many partners, something she hadn't ever given herself the permission to do. She was now able to state her intentions and needs clearly to all her sexual partners, inform them of the "deal," and get them on board: Sex without attachments or commitment. Show up, have sex, and that is it.

In our last conversation, she was contemplating moving into a more committed relationship with one of them, but it was very clear to her: having "physical sex" with multiple partners had been a really healing period for her. It allowed her to have her own sexual revolution. She needed to indulge in it. She felt the freedom to explore what she liked, experience different sensations with multiple partners, and operate outside of the framework of attachment. It was liberating.

Although Sacha was aware that non-attachment is a form of avoidance from further emotional pain, she needed to experience this phase of sexual exploration for herself, to feel the pleasure of sexuality in her body, enjoy being desired without any other burdens. Having multiple partners freed something up for her instead of zooming in on one person and loading the relationship with expectations. She was also aware that at some point, the natural progression would lead to a deepening intimacy with someone. Yet the healing came from granting herself permission to experience and indulge in it, knowing that when she was ready, she would open to something more.

Sacha's story gives us insight into how simple, straightforward physical sex can be very healing. To decide what we want and to give ourselves permission to do it is empowering and may be the exact thing we need at the moment. In Chapter Eleven, we will further explore different practices of mindfulness to bring you toward better inhabiting your body.

Soul Reverb

Now that we've explored physical sex and its usefulness, it's time for reflection. Get your workbook or journal and write down your answers.

1. To what degree are you present in your body? Can you easily surrender to your bodily sensations, to pleasure? Are you present to what goes on for your body? What is your degree of "body" mindfulness?
2. Do you feel any shame around your body and/or weight, body hair, body shape, shape or length of genitalia? Describe the shame that comes up.
3. Do you feel any shame in letting your sexual energy freely express itself in your body? Why?
4. What part of the shame that you carry are you willing to let go of today? Discover what it is.

Chapter Affirmations

- When I am present in my body, I am at home.
- I thrive when I am present to my body.
- My body knows when it's safe and when it isn't.
- My body needs love, care, and kindness.

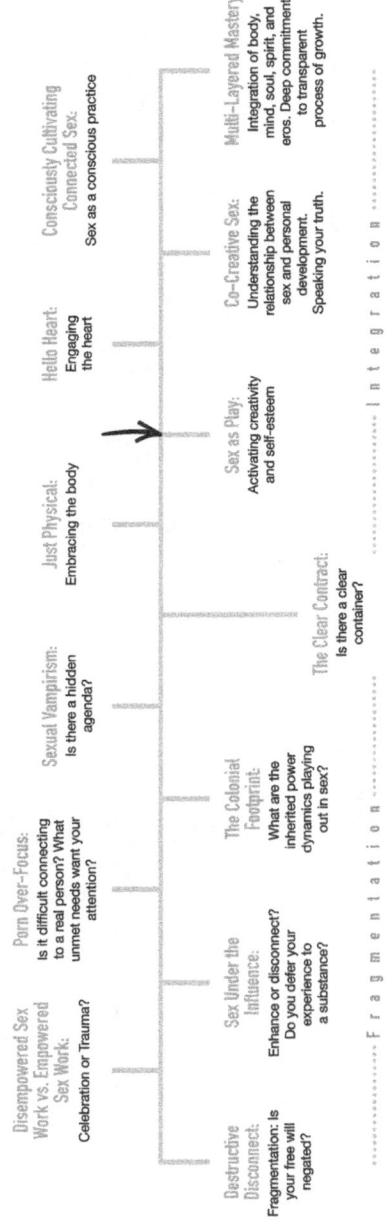

CHAPTER 8:

TIME TO PLAY

"Physics is like sex: sure, it may give some practical results, but that's not why we do it."

—Richard Feynman

"Today, make time to play."

—Na'ama Yehuda

"Forget about sex. Just play first. Dance, sing, read to each other, breathe together—communicate. Don't count on sex to be the door to intimacy. It's the other way around: first develop intimacy skills. Then make love to enjoy them."

—Margot Anand

When offering live workshops, "activating" play for participants thrills me. Something happens in the room: it goes from serious stiffness to suddenly palpable aliveness. Participants get an experience of stepping into "freedom." They get to try something that goes beyond their habitual and familiar everyday self. They can explore various facets of themselves they might not know how to otherwise access. Play is a portal to the unexplored self.

I created an amusing game that I named the "Animal Love" game. Initially, I had no idea if adults would go for it! Was it too silly? I tested it out one evening and it was an instant hit, which shows me how eager we are as humans to indulge in play.

I told the participants to pair up with someone in the group and I called out various animals. The game involved becoming the animal by imagining its seduction techniques. I'll never forget all these seemingly serious adults relaxing into warbling turkeys, dancing snakes, fighting tigers, and, yes, the unforgettable mating bullfrog. In every corner of the room, there was laughter, movement, and play.

Connection and joy were palpable. Participants who initially seemed shy and unexpressed suddenly were accessing shared delight and outrageous interpretations. The game revealed a more magnetic and charming way of being, the kind of person you would want to frolic in bed with. I was in a state of tearful hilarity the whole time. The game created immediate relatedness and playfulness.

This is the tremendous potential of play.

In this chapter you will:

- Explore the potential of play
- Define the qualities of play
- Experience Maria's story with Ecstatic Play
- Discover Seani Love's story with Conscious Kink

Section 1. Expanding Play

When we think play, we automatically think children. But truly, it is a way of being that involves being carefree, generating possibilities, and joy. Who doesn't like a playful banter? Who doesn't feel charmed by a creative mind? Play is the next space to explore on the sex continuum.

By adding "play" to physical sex, we access a whole new level of connection and possibilities. Here, we activate our soul life, comprised of our feeling and thought life. At the most basic level, we have sex as play with "no-strings-attached." Each person involved holds an authentic foundation of respect and concern for the other's well-being, a desire to explore and create, genuine openness, without necessarily having any deeper feelings—just yet. Each person desires to share pleasure and enjoy the present moment. Here, the line has been clearly drawn: no commitment, just amusement. When both people agree to this, and clarity reigns, room opens for light and playful sex. This is a little bit more involved than simple "genital rubbing," since trust and mutual respect invite sharing and imagination.

Self-interest becomes replaced with getting into someone's else's world, sharing each other's imaginations. The lightheartedness tells us the heart is present, albeit it in a free-spirited way. It is all fun and play—and stays that way. And this may take on many creative forms. People may want to playfully romp, take on roles, enact fantasies, and play out games. They may have fun with sex toys. Basically, they get creative with each other.

Now, bring that to the bedroom. It doesn't take much, and yet it can completely change the whole sexual experience and access to connection with your partner.

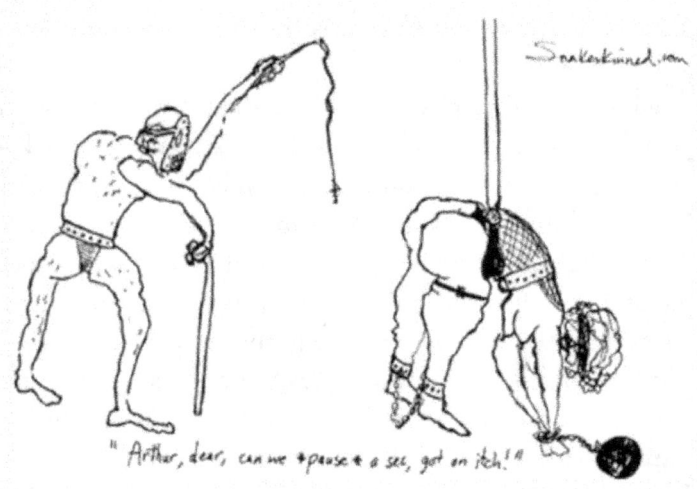

When children play, they are fully engaged. What's more, everything is possible. Imagine a child building a sandcastle: children are fully present to their creation. When playing cops and robbers, they run with fullness of heart. They fully embody the authority of the policeman, the secrecy of the robber. I still remember the feelings I had when playing "Star Wars" as a child. Since we were two girls amongst a slew of boys, we made up that we were "Princess Leia Twins." The swing was our spaceship. For children, everything seems possible. A spoon can become a phone, then a musical instrument, then a telescope. You can be a pirate, then a princess, then a prisoner. The story unfolds in real-time. How much permission do you give yourself to live out that potential? To play with it? To go where you may have never been?

When you engage in sex as play, you are letting your creative self out of the sack to have fun and explore possibilities. Is your creative self alive and well, or is it stifled, a little rigid? Do you become passive? Do you need to control? Do you live into your imaginations or do you cut them short?

Can you actually give yourself permission to play and have fun? Or are you limited by pragmatic considerations, what ifs? Are you always on a tight timeline? Is sex contained to a strict protocol? Do you let that inner child go wild, or is it bound by conventions, by unconscious roles or rules? How free are you to let possibilities unfold? How much magic are you willing to let in?

Imagine two people on stage in a game of improvisation. They are given a topic and must create something together. Think about how comfortable they might be in pulling the unknown into the present, the unformed into form, the unimagined into action. Look at whether they are capable of fully living into what emerges, if they withhold, are tentative, or if they jump in powerfully? Imagine one person feeling at ease, and the other discomfort. One comes across powerfully, the other awkward.

What makes their experiences of improvisation different? The first person has permission to be. The other doesn't claim the same right. With self-assurance, you fill out any character, any storyline, and you feel safe to reveal those tender spaces. You allow yourself to be seen, to take up space. You surrender yourself to the game. If you lack confidence, your voice falls back. You shrink. You look uncomfortable, which will also be perceived by the audience. Awkwardness comes from deep-seated insecurities that push you off kilter. In turn, confidence allows you to show up with a much larger scope of possibilities.

Tools for Play

You may hear voices in your head saying, "No, you can't do that," or "That is not how we behave" or "That is not proper." Perhaps: "That is just weird." Maybe you hear, "Oh, you are not good enough! You don't deserve this!" Maybe you feel the embarrassment of performing and hear: "I don't know what the heck I'm doing!" You can start flagging this internal voice as your conditioning.

But let's be clear for sex: there is a big difference between not giving yourself permission to play and listening to your gut tell you that you are crossing a boundary you don't want to cross. It's important to appreciate the difference.

Giving yourself permission to have boundaries is what makes playing safe. When you play, there are all kinds of rules by which the playing parties abide in order to keep the game fun. If you start breaking all the rules to a card game or a board game, chances are the other players are going to get mad. But once the parameters are established, your capacity to play is also your capacity for freedom.

Other restraints may appear here: your self-esteem, confidence, and power. If you lack confidence, your play will be tentative or perhaps even passive. I think we can all agree that the creative quotient and synergy drops if someone is passive or withdraws.

As an example: smitten with tango in my thirties, I hired a talented teacher to give me some private lessons. He was very attuned to every move I made and could offer perceptive feedback. In tango, like in most couples dancing, there is the leader and the person led, aka follower.

In this specific situation, I was being led, and I paid careful attention to his lead and executed without resistance.

I thought I was being a good dancer by "responding" immediately to his lead. But in fact, that was not the case. "No. This makes for a very BORING dance," he said. He took my hand and told me to put presence in that hand, to put up some resistance. He needed to feel my presence there or else it would be like dancing with a vaporous curtain. Who wants to dance with a ghost? To understand this opened my eyes up to fascinating dynamics playing out.

He explained that when I presented some resistance, I communicated to him that I was an integral part of the creative process. He gets inspired by his partner's energy. That informs what happens in the dance. Most of all, it brings energy to the dance and tremendous creative potential. In fact, it quickens response time because pressure allows for connection.

In sex as play, you will be exploring these various dynamics for yourself too. Can you fill out your space as in a dance? It will help you discover your edges when it comes to your capacity to engage, to own yourself, to initiate, imagine, create, and generate playful and fun synergy.

If we contrast physical and playful sex, we are breathing in a whole new dimension of aliveness, laughter, and joy. You will notice how free you are with your inner child, if it needs nurturing, or if it needs to be given permission to play just a little more whole-heartedly. It will show you your edges, where you need to give yourself permission, where you hold back, where you become stiff and passive. Sex is adult play. Here, you start to experience yourself as a creator.

Let's experience some Ecstatic Play with Maria Palumbo.

Maria Palumbo's Story—Ecstatic Play

I'll introduce Maria more extensively in chapter 11. For now, let's just blindly follow her on the trails of her playful night of sensual passion that she summoned then ushered into ecstatic existence for herself.

It was her birthday week and she was ready for adventure. Being in an open marriage, her sensual forays are endorsed and encouraged by her husband. "He actually loves how sexually alive I am. He tells me I am so connected to myself; not everyone has that, you know!" She packed her bag with a change of clothes, not sure what would unfold at the creative evening of Ecstatic Dance. Before leaving, she set an intention: She wanted magic and adventure.

The room was full of bodies in movement, unleashed to rhythm, internalizing sensation, embracing self-expression. Maria found herself dancing with a man. Their bodies moved together, hand movements were intentional on legs, on neck. It was arousing, not from the standpoint of her genitalia, but from that of her whole being. Sweat overflowed, became indistinct: *mine, his?* No matter: They were simply drenched in this water. They were moving in it. There wasn't any focus on genitalia, it was simply the enjoyment of this respectful erotic dance, movement, and worship of each other's presence.

Maria was left breathless. Sweat was everywhere. Once it was over, she needed to be with herself. In the past, she would have needed to seek something out, like that person. She would have needed to talk to him. Maybe even ask herself: what did I just do? But in that moment, she felt complete. All she needed was to be quiet, still. She drank a glass of water. Cooled down.

She became aware of her skin: sensuality made it feel thinner, more sensitive. All her senses were awake. She was letting the rush of energy settle down. She was aware of how gentle she needed to be with herself after such an opening experience. She needed to downshift, to slow down. She held a space of kindness for herself.

What was that!? she contemplated. It was such an intense experience, all she wanted to do at that moment was integrate it. Breathe into it, appreciate its gifts. Relish it. She stood in her body, feeling delicious in her own pleasure. She thought, *I can go home now. I am complete.*

Then a man brushed past her. He walked past her then turned around and locked eyes with her for thirty seconds then walked towards her. They were nose to nose for about forty-five minutes, breathing, only touching lightly, and both enjoying the eroticism of the energy pulsating between them. Barely anything was happening, there was a stillness, and yet, Maria found herself moaning, then laughing, at times holding onto him, then letting go. "It felt like my energy was water and someone had met me there in water, which made it that much more sensual, gentle, and intoxicating for me."

Maria loves the feeling of energy pulling between two bodies without needing to close in on it. "I like making space for that pulsating energy between two bodies," she says. At that point, they had barely embraced; at most, their tongues touched, quickly grazed, and that simple flicker of the tongue shot a current of bliss up her body. "It is because we had slowed down, that's what made it feel so good. I was very aware of every little inch, and every little breath that he gave me."

Maria shares that his energy was in this powerful masculine place, and he was unwavering. "His energy was so calm and contained, so held, it was easy for me to meet him there." His presence helped her drop into her own calmness. "His touch was so grounding and yet so intoxicating; I didn't want to let go. I knew I was complete, there was no one else I wanted to connect with, nobody else I wanted to talk to."

And after that, he looked at her and said: "Do you want to go on an adventure?"

Maria responded: "Yesss please!"

From that moment on, the whole night played out in this space of erotic bliss, the sharing of bodily fluids, laughter, heart connection, silliness, and sex, all in the container of practicing safer sex. There was depth too: the kind that can only come from when you've just met someone. "The easy kind of depth where you can be really free because you have no attachment to who that person is to you, or if they are going to like what you say," she says. There is a quality of timelessness and freedom that is gifted in these moments.

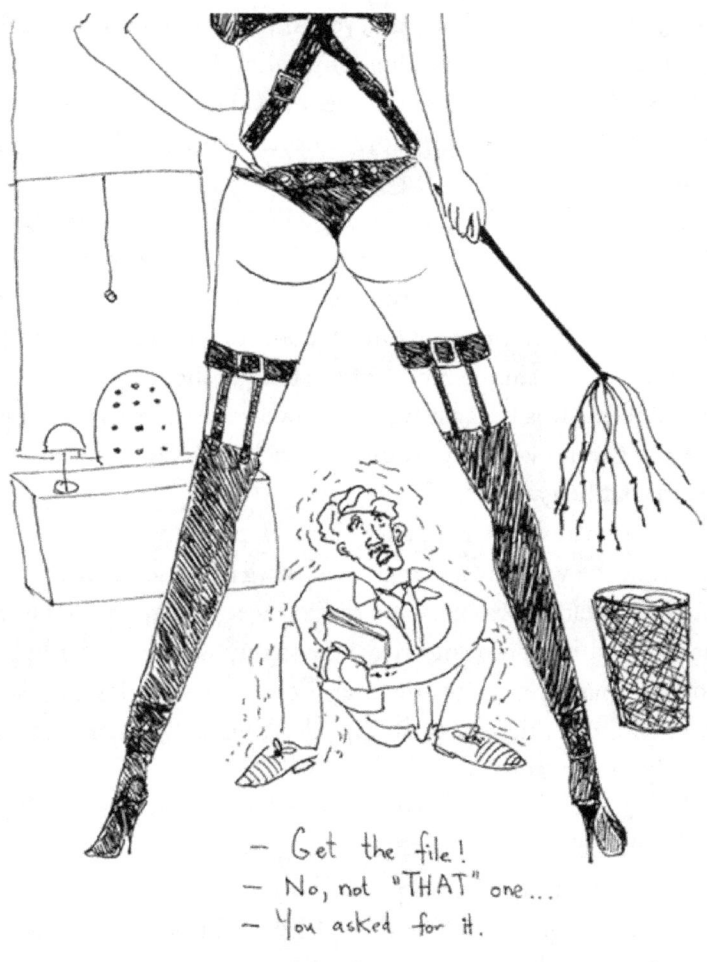

The Pleasure of Decluttering

Maria let us in on this sensual adventure where sex is essentially light, playful, creative, fun, and healthy. You may have your own version of this. You may recognize some of these elating qualities and sensations as your own. After such an experience, you can recognize that your body feels refreshed and good. Your energy fields and those of your partner are mutually nourished and enlivened. During this period of exploration, potential and genuine reciprocal interest are present. It fills you with energy and aliveness. In contrast with Sexual Vampirism, there is no drop or loss of energy, nor sense of discomfort after it's finished. Such experiences can feel almost contained in another realm. Once they are finished, most often, they are complete. Unless a relationship is ignited!

Section 2. Surprise! Kinky Play can Heal You

"Your pain is the breaking of the shell that encloses your understanding."

—Khalil Gibran

Before I talk about "Conscious Kink," let me define how people use the word kink in popular culture. It is referred to as "unusual taste in sexual behavior." "Conscious Kink" involves establishing a conscious context for the behavior. The process is driven by intentionality and respect, rather than indulging in gratuitous behavior for the sake of it.

As we progress across the Continuum of Connection, "Conscious Kink" can be understood as a subcategory of fun and playful sex with a kinky twist. It may not be light-hearted since it usually involves consciously playing with sensitive trigger points held in the body and soul. Here, you may be using play to experience a cathartic release, which will most likely involve tears. Since we are entering higher-stake games, potentially unleashing important unprocessed energies, a solid and safe container is essential. The people holding the container must have the capacity to hold these strong emotional releases and powerful energies to avoid re-traumatizing the people involved. Emotional tsunamis are real.

So here, when playing with powerful forces and potential pent-up trauma, you need a solid grounding in yourself. While it's certainly exciting, you need the emotional maturity to avoid further fragmenting yourself and your partner. The difference between unhelpful and helpful kink is whether the sexual experiences and games reinforce fragmentation of the people involved or if they allow for integration.

Alternatively, if further attachment to your pain points occur because you are enjoying the pay-off, instead of transmuting them, this behavior is ultimately self-sabotaging: you are deepening your state of fragmentation, meaning your growth as a person stagnates because you've created a glitch in the system, a negative self-reinforcing loop that keeps your energy from flowing freely.

Our sexual energy is a heightened flow of life forces, or "chi," blasting through our body—which will be better grasped when addressed in the context of conscious practices of sexuality such as tantra, or Taoism. This powerful flow is constantly seeking to integrate your whole being. Energy wants to flow. It doesn't like getting stuck behind a dam. Our emotional blocks and glitches create blocks to the energy flow in our bodies. A river is meant to lead you to the ocean, whereas your sexual energy leads you to wholeness. Anything damming up the natural process would necessarily lead to some form of uncomfortable healing crisis.

Let's discover "Conscious Kink" with Seani Love's story—the master—and how higher-stake games can allow you to further your process of integration.

Seani Love's Story—Guiding Kinky Healing

I discovered Seani Love in the ever-tightening web of social media. A social media contact of mine in the UK had been to one of his workshops in England and was raving about him on Instagram, saying, "I love this man." Being a sex educator, her interest tweaked mine and I started following his posts and witnessing his journey. He would give glimpses of his workshops across Europe, an article in the UK *Sunday Times* weekend magazine and *Cosmopolitan* showcasing him as a male escort, and his walk across the red carpet at the Berlinale International Film Festival where *Touch Me Not* was awarded the Golden Bear for Best Film in 2018. This is a film in which he plays a BDSM male escort. Clearly, Seani Love is on a roll.

In 2015, Seani was joint winner of Sex Worker of the Year award for his activism and work in overcoming the collective sexual challenges of our time, which is an award granted by the Sexual Freedom Awards in the UK, a show of recognition from his peers. But what struck me most was how authentic Seani would come across on his posts. No artifices, simply him, showing up, authentically speaking about his sex work and educational workshops on the themes of Conscious Kink and Shadow Tantra—terms he uses to communicate what he does.

Communication is essential in his field, of course, and he is well aware of this. Misconceptions and misrepresentation of BDSM and sex work are frequent, so I was pleased when he accepted my request for an interview. His work is rooted in ethical considerations. His communication style is grounded and straightforward. I felt he was the perfect guide to bring us into the darker sides of our psyche and show how playing them out within the context of sexuality could be powerfully cathartic and healing for the people involved.

Seani Love chose this path because he had always been very kinky himself and yet experienced a tremendous amount of shame because of it. From the time of his burgeoning teenage sexuality, he would have strange desires and impulses that were not socially acceptable, including choking someone or consensual non-consent rape fantasies. He couldn't really understand what was going on with him; these impulses didn't seem quite normal and would surface deep feelings of shame, which he imagines compares to how a gay person would feel to coming out. The shame can be overwhelming. The fear of being misunderstood and vilified can be soul-crushing.

In his mid-thirties, as he partook in introspective exercises in a counseling program, he recognized the origin of his impulses. When he had reached puberty, between the ages of fourteen and sixteen, he felt incredibly horny, full of lust, and yet had to suppress it all. He also recognized how needy he was to simply be loved. Being a young heterosexual man, his lust couldn't be met by the girls of his age, and with hindsight, he understands why.

In the normative heterosexual gender binary model, all kinds of negative messaging were given to young women, including slut-shaming for having or wanting sex. Even if they did fancy him, they simply wouldn't go there for fear of being rejected, ostracized, called-out, and shamed. Seani recalls constantly being rejected, the experience of many boys of his generation. "I felt I had a big heart, I really just wanted to be loved, and I had a high sex drive." He resorted to a lot of masturbation. This frustration led his masturbatory fantasies into various scenarios of forced sexual activity. "My fantasies at that time would involve the idea that I was going to rape someone, choke them, overpower them, and beat them. And, in the process, they were going to fall in love with me."

His life changed when he actually started having intercourse with women. As it turned out, one of his lovers had been sexually assaulted in a way very similar to his fantasies. It had been a devastating experience for her, and her whole body would freeze up when they became sexual. Seani, interested in ritual and various shamanic practices, recreated her trauma within a healing ritual they designed to help her overcome it. Together, they retraced the steps of where her trauma happened and replayed it, but this time as consciously as they possibly could to find the exact point when the trauma locked into her body.

"She would micromanage me. She would tell me what way to stand and how to hold her, and what words to use, when to rewind it a little, until we found the exact point." Seani needed to remain aware while unleashing his menacing, predatorial energy so he could be really present with her. Seani was fully in his evil beast mode: he was holding her down, naked, drooling, snarling, and aggressively telling her what he was going to do to her. He had alcohol on his breath and was knocking her against a surface while speaking the words she instructed him to use. She would say: "Say this word, use this word, not that word."

"Today," Seani explained, "we would have safe words to navigate that, but back then, we didn't have those words. The whole purpose of the ritual was for her to tell me those things." She couldn't move. She had frozen up, her legs held apart by the pressure of his hands. Yet at one moment, her body suddenly unthawed. Her whole body unfroze, a sort of loosening out.

In that moment, Seani shifted too; while he held the same physical pressure on her body, he stopped with the snarling and let his empathy kick in. This allowed her to release a significant amount of tension, followed by long, deep sobs. Seani simply held her for a long time until she felt completely soothed. "This was a really amazing moment in my life," says Seani. "It set her free." But not only was this a tremendous breakthrough for her, it was for Seani as well. "It was healing for me too because of all the shame I had around my sex, my desires, my dark fantasies. 'Your kink that you're ashamed of,' she said, 'is actually medicine for the world. What you think is your burden is actually your medicine, go out and share it with the world.'" In a sacred and highly consensual container, this darker play could be helpful to others. This turned out to be a profound revelation for Seani.

After this potent experience, Seani decided to start learning and exploring kink more proactively. One of his favorite authors, teachers, and muses is Raven Kaldera, teacher of BDSM spirituality and much more. When Raven came to London from the US, Seani organized his workshop, which included participants from as far away as Prague. Subsequently, Seani agreed to go to a workshop in Prague where he was asked for a private session. This launched him as a workshop leader, a sex educator, a private sex worker, and healing catalyst for countless women and men.

Seani clarifies that he works with people of all identified genders, yet as a heterosexual man, he can only offer arousal services for women, which, he notes, is never offered on the first session. He follows two threads in his workshops. For one, he teaches how to navigate consent and boundaries in real-time, a much-needed skill in our era of sexual emancipation and the #MeToo movement. He explains that this is not something he learned growing up, and he teaches how to ask for consent gracefully, how to say no in an empowered way, and how to accept it without feeling rejected. As in any game, there are rules that need to be negotiated so the partners can fully enjoy the ride. This is true for sex as play, and even more so when the "play" unleashes powerful shadow characters into the unfolding plot, as happens with BDSM.

With the second workshop thread, he teaches participants to hold space for their sexual partners, not dissimilar to how a therapist would create a safe healing space for their clients to process emotions. In the BDSM world, he explores with his participants the how-to's to create a healthy container for the person taking on the journey.

Seani Love is well aware that accidents can happen and that in the BDSM world it is possible to re-traumatize yourself or your sexual partner, which is why it requires careful navigation. It is also possible to get in a self-reinforcing loop; instead of releasing the trauma, you can get attached to it and want to replay it, over and over again. He cites Susan David's work on why and how people process emotions.[21] Some people just stir it around, some people release it. But to release the patterns or dynamics of trauma, you have to make a conscious decision.

Seani believes "it is the same thing for dark, erotic fantasies: you can bathe, wade and soak in them, feel them, but not release them. But with some consciousness, you can release them, which sets you free." He is also aware that not everyone entering the journey will break the erotic loop, meaning if they are attached to the pleasure pay off instead of transmuting the source of the pain itself, you can develop a fixation. For his part, he knows he has addressed his own teenage years. He is aware that his fantasies are still present and strong, but he has consciously made them his allies instead.

He also adds that it is important for him not to judge people who simply want to get off on their darker fantasies. Shame is not a helpful emotion in moving forward. He says, "If you like a spanking, and I give you one, and it is not part of a healing journey and you simply like it, we don't need to judge that. Sometimes a spanking can be amazingly healing in itself. But there is no need to judge the person even though it is not part of a healing journey."

Nevertheless, Seani's main thrust in his sessions are designed for exploring consciousness and personal growth. It's about finding what is there. "It's about becoming super aware that there are many possibilities. Some mainstream BDSM tropes dictate ideas such

---

21 David, Susan. (2016) Emotional Agility: Get Unstuck, Embrace Change, and Thrive in Work and Life. Penguin Random House.

as the top is always the sadist who decides everything, whereas the bottom is always the one on the receiving end. Another common idea is that the masochist is expected to behave in certain, largely predictable ways. As we become more conscious, we can let those tropes fall away in favor of one of the many other ways to behave and dividing up the roles."

Seani isn't interested in participating in dark fantasies that are just "horrible for the sake of being horrible." Rather, he is looking for a sense of redemption at the end of the journey. Just as with his initial partner, the reenactment of her trauma allowed her to rewrite the script of her story, which ultimately freed her from it. He has helped other clients regress back to childhood in order to re-enact scenes in which they were too young to say no. The re-enactment allows them to re-write the ending of their story and reclaim their right to have boundaries and a voice.

Sexuality is Seani's gateway, but his work is much more than that. He wants his clients to experience both their emotional body and their potential. Seani's approach is inspired by Carl Jung's work on the process of individuation[22]: finding your divine purpose, experiencing your true will, and embodying your true self. By exploring the various archetypes within you, you become aware of what is playing out within your life.

His healing journeys have benefitted many. He can guide his clients on journeys that deal with everything from trauma to daddy issues, which he says could be a whole career unto itself, or simply allowing his clients to have the true "boyfriend" experiences of cuddling, love, and passionate sex. On Seani's path of self-mastery, he has learned how to access true love by consciously opening his heart during his sessions.

"I can fall madly in love with a client, which is initiatory for them as well. It is to become super aware of what is happening on

---

22 http://journalpsyche.org/jung-and-his-individuation-process/

an energy level. The heart reaches out, it commits to being in love, it reaches out and attaches. We entwine, cuddle each other, and at the end of the session, come back to self, with no attachments nor dependency on either of us." He notes that some women don't want a boyfriend, but want to feel that nourishment of love, feel loved, and then go on with their busy lives.

Other women come to him to access their sexual power. In fact, one of his regular clients would come for overnight sessions once a month to access her "wild sexuality." Seani uses a map of different personas described by Jung to access different archetypes. They are designed to open the treasure trove of his client's psyche and try on various masks.

Seani also facilitates healing around female rage and male shame. He tells me of a woman who hired him to help her access her rage around catcalling and inappropriate touch. After pre-negotiating boundaries and being clear with what he was going to do, he would start taunting and jostling her, making inappropriate comments while gazing at her body in sexualized ways. By locking fingers with him and pushing up against him, she managed to unleash her pent-up anger towards the male gaze.

Her frustration had been growing over the years, trapped in places such as her belly, womb, and sexual organs. She had never had a chance to express to the men her deep-seated frustrations. In the session, she finally let them loose: "You disgust me, you fucking bastard," she said along with more fury that bubbled up from the session. "It was a really beautiful moment," says Seani, who also acknowledges that it is edgy work for him, as he is accessing a part that exists in him, and yet does so only with clear consent.

Seani also supports men who feel completely sexually disempowered, often in reaction to expressions of toxic masculinity. At an early age, these men may have been disconnected from both their heart and sexuality, just as he had been: shoulders hunched over, "cocks shriveled". Locking fingers, they battle strength back into the disempowered men, allowing them to will their sexuality and fierceness back into existence. Instead of repressing that part of themselves, they are given permission to embody it, express it.

Seani Love's treasure trove is vast and rich, and when opened, it can take his clients on tremendous journeys filled with powerful, colorful experiences to explore their consciousness, their emotional body, and their scope for pleasure while simultaneously healing very deep wounds that have haunted some clients from as far back as preverbal stages of their development, meaning before they could even talk.

Seani's key to success is by creating the proper container for his clients. He achieves this through ritual and clear intentions, through setting absolute boundaries and creating a safe space for the mystery to reveal itself.

Another element of Seani's success is his policy of protecting his clients. As soon as they realize discomfort, he urges them to let him know, regardless of the lapsed time. He wants to build solid and safe boundaries for their physical, emotional, mental, and spiritual safety. Both these skills—boundary setting and holding space—go a long way in creating the right conditions for his conscious kink and shadow tantra to be powerful tools for consciousness and healing.

Soul Reverb

Now that you see sex as play, even kinky play, it's time for reflection. Reach for your workbook or journal and jot down your answers.

1. How much permission do you give yourself to play, explore, discover? Can you surrender to the game? Do you need to control everything? Do you have a habit of raining on the fun parade?
2. Do you know how to navigate giving yourself permission to explore and having the necessary conversation about rules

and boundaries that address your needs? Can you do this without the guilt factor?
3. How attentive are you to the dynamics playing out? When looking at the dynamics you put yourself in, what do you discover about yourself? How can you play with your shadow to give it expression?

Chapter Affirmations

- When I let my inner child play, I experience freedom.
- Healthy boundaries and a solid container allow for integration.
- When I show up with confidence, I generate potential.
- Consciously playing with my shadow makes me whole.

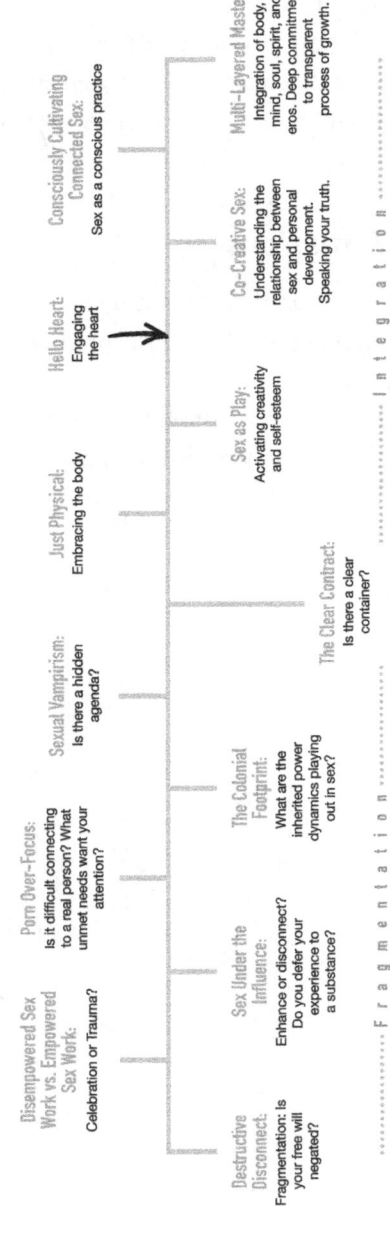

CHAPTER 9:

REMOVE THE ARMOR

"Love is a fire. But whether it is going to warm your hearth or burn down your house, you can never tell."
—Joan Crawford

"To me, obligation is not love. Letting someone be open, honest, and free—that's love. It's got to come natural and it's got to be real."
—Dolly Parton

"When you fish for love, bait with your heart, not your brain."
—Mark Twain, Notebook, 1898

As love grows, sex becomes less and less motivated by self-interest. There is a desire to give to the other person as opposed to simply taking. It also involves being capable of receiving someone's love. The interesting thing is that even though you are in love with someone, you may have a habit of disconnecting from your heart during sex since it takes vulnerability to bring your presence, love, and care to your partner. This can be quite scary and intimidating. When we bring the heart into sex, another level of connection is present. Observe what happens to the quality of the meeting and exchange. What happens when you look into each other's eyes? Do you feel your heart? Is there a tingling feeling? Is there a flood of deep reverence?

When you involve the heart in sex, you access a whole new dimension in the relationship and sexual experience. Not only are you physically involved, but your deepest emotions are engaged as well. Opening the heart means your actions are guided by a genuine, heartfelt interest in the other person. In her book *Shake Your Soul Song*, Devi Ward refers to love as "the joy of bringing happiness and pleasure to the other person." With the heart involved, we are not purely motivated by our self-interest; we are compelled by love for the other person as a multi-layered individual. We develop a much deeper connection and respect for them, their integrity, and their feelings, as well as care for their body.

In this chapter you will:

- Discover love as a force
- Notice what is under your heart's armor
- Explore why we avoid feeling
- Read Charlie's story of unleashing sensual sex

Opening up one's heart is not necessarily an easy thing to do; in fact, it is challenging for most people. You need to pass through the initiation of vulnerability, which requires your soul's bulldog—the lower ego—to heel. The bulldog barks out of fear of feeling: "Keep those feelings far away from my heart!" By keeping feelings at bay, you avoid pain. You protect yourself. But when you cut yourself off from your heart, there are consequences as well: you lose out on giving and receiving love.

To open your heart means that you enter a place of vulnerability, where you strive to be authentic, to reveal yourself, and to be truthful about what you feel. This involves surrendering to acknowledging what's actually going on for you. Let me share one powerful experience I had that totally blew me open and helped me reconcile the vulnerabilities of the heart.

I had been working on myself intensely, restoring myself back from pain—relationships being a difficult theme in my life—when I was struck by a new acquaintance. A gush of energy overtook my body. I tried ignoring the feeling, suppressing it, pretending it wasn't there, pushing it away like I had done many times in the past, trying to protect myself from the vagaries of the heart, but alas, this time I could no longer control it. I was already wide open; there was no going back. But I didn't want him to know. *What if he doesn't love me back!? That would be sooo hard on my feeling of self-worth!!* Rejection. OUCHHH! So, after a session with my massage therapist, I dared sharing with her what was going on in my buoyant soul life. "It's like this love is coming into me and it's BIG! It's like this FORCE that is taking hold of my body and I can't control it!" I said with resignation as tears trickled down my face.

She said, "That, right there, that is You. That is your capacity to love." Instantly, her words appeased me. My breath changed. I didn't need to control it anymore. It was "my" love. It had nothing to do with this particular person. He was the spark, but the love, that was mine, it was my capacity to love, and there was nothing to be ashamed of! I didn't need to block it out anymore; I could just let it come in and nourish me. I could allow myself to bathe in it, simply enjoy this depth of feeling that I was accessing. I was this teary-eyed puppy suddenly realizing how good life felt. What I understood was that my open heart was now ripe to channel that love. It was ready to feel again.

It was deeply liberating to stop trying to control the heart and to give myself permission to feel. It actually takes a lot of energy to resist and block this force, a contortion act, really! I am well

Remove the Armor

aware that opening the heart is challenging for many, particularly if they are afraid of getting hurt. The more I deepen my work, the more I realize this is the case for most people. We are all hurt from something! It could be from previous heartaches with lovers, but it extends to all relations. Sometimes people are aching from their own family systems or impactful life experiences. Feeling of abandonment, rejection, criticism, betrayal, bullying, you name it—will impact your willingness to open your heart back up. Who wants to feel that again? It's downright painful. That is why shielding and numbing become so appealing. And yet, so costly as well. Cutting out love from your life generates deep loneliness that can, as it grows, lead to unfortunate circumstances.

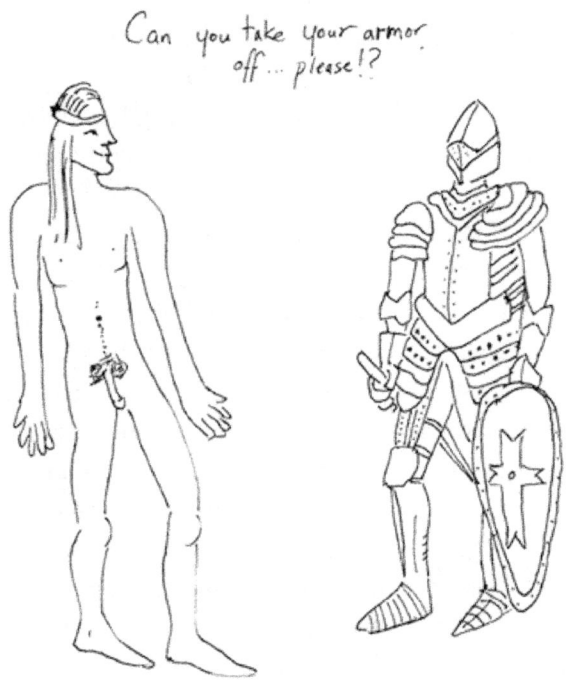

In order to access love once more, you must reach beyond your coping mechanisms. This means following the traces of your shadow and catching yourself in the act: what do you do to avoid feeling? Where do you hide? How do you harden yourself? What and who do you cut out of your life to survive? Retrace where these habits come from, identify the pain that activated them. What is blocking coming to terms with that situation?

Then, you need to remind yourself that this comes from the past and that it is safe to feel again. Once you manage to drop your coping mechanisms, the returns are tremendous.

Allowing yourself to feel your emotions, instead of negating or repressing them, allows for more depth in the experience and more fulfilling sex. But, simultaneously, it also involves discovering your fears and wounds, and working through them. This is a necessary rite of passage on this path to the integrated human being.

Charlie's Story—Unleashing Sensual Sex

Charlie is a brilliant artist and now mother to a toddler. She is stunning, with a long, curly mane of black locks, bright, intelligent eyes, and olive skin. When we first got acquainted, I noticed she had this cold and heady way about her, which contrasted with her lush looks. Seemingly her masculine side was very present: she was pragmatic, down to earth, a gets-the-job-done type of person with solid and clear unemotional boundaries. Yet it felt like something was being held back; her sensual femininity was suppressed. She spoke from a place of straight-forward rationality. Her husband, on the other hand, had much more receptive energy. He was introverted, sensitive, more of the bookish-type.

They would often joke that she was the husband and he the wife. The issue they were dealing with was that while they were the best friends in the world, she wasn't feeling any sexual desire for him. This was, of course, distressing for both. I should add that this feeling was probably exacerbated by the fact that she had given birth to a daughter, and her energies were used for the feeding and the tending of their child's needs. Regardless, Charlie also knew there was more to it.

In her sessions, we discovered that she grew up witnessing a toxic relationship between her mother and father. To put it bluntly, she said: "My dad was a real jerk to my mom." He would put her down, say mean things to her, mock her ideas, and make her look ridiculous on a regular basis. The mother did not have an empowering context in which to express herself. She was always at risk of being emotionally maimed and was dominated by her husband's harsh and critical behavior.

Charlie, being a very smart little girl, saw who had the upper hand in this dynamic, who wielded the power, and how to behave if she wanted to avoid experiencing the same types of put-downs. It pained her to watch his cruelty, but it also had become a surprisingly normal part of the family culture.

Her father's behavior made "feeling" a risky affair in the household; the toll on her mother was a plummeting self-esteem. Despite his treatment of her mother, Charlie says her father didn't treat her in the same way. She had learned to play the game right; she learned to stay clear of any emotional vulnerability, and essentially she controlled herself. Unconsciously, Charlie didn't want to run the risk of being treated like her mother. This is how she started shutting down her feminine side, because apparently it was a sign of weakness. If she lived in the space of the feminine, perhaps she too would be treated in a demeaning way.

In this hostile landscape it wasn't safe to express the tenderness and vulnerabilities of the heart. Better to override her feelings, stay pragmatic, and dull the heart. As a tender young girl, seeing her mother treated with such harshness was a very painful experience. In fact, throughout her life Charlie always felt compelled to stick up for the underdog. If she saw a situation where someone was being bullied or mistreated, she was called to stick up for them. And yet she also concedes that growing up at home, Charlie would never speak up against her father to protect her mom. She just endured the situation.

Charlie also admitted to watching herself becoming somewhat of a steamroller to her partner at times. She would shut him down, criticize him or dismiss him. "And I know he's had his own trauma, so I actually can't believe I'm doing this!" she said.

Before this relationship, she was always the one in charge, setting the pace, the one calling the shots, and the one ending relationships. But she chuckled as she shared with me that in one relationship, she found herself expressing herself in unfamiliar feminine ways. She never wore skirts or spent time putting on makeup. But being sexy was now a great concern to her, and she was really eager to please him. She fell under a powerful spell, and the pull was strong. She deeply yearned for his approval, and yet his treatment of her was poor, at times unpleasant. This was the first time she felt she had surrendered the reins and allowed herself to express her femininity. When he finally dismissed her and they broke up, it shattered her sense of self. It also confirmed her programming: when you show up in the feminine, you are ill-treated, put down, and eventually dismissed.

As we deepened our session, I asked her to reconnect to the moments where her mother was being bullied and to feel what her mom endured. This was challenging for her. Part of her strategy to survive had been to shut it completely out and avoid feeling it. I asked her to get out of her head and drop into her heart and feel her mother's pain. Charlie recognized a lot of sadness, feelings of unworthiness, and feeling small.

Little did she know that her rational mind had been her hideout: there she didn't actually have to feel her mother's pain. She didn't have to be burdened with the constant assault on her own sensitivity.

In alienating parts of our being, we end up limiting our life as well. As Charlie allowed herself to feel for her mother, she also had a better access to what her beau could be feeling too. As her new understanding took hold on her life, she told me she had started seeing new dimensions in her husband, and that she suddenly found herself admiring him. She started noticing when she would retreat into her head and why. She started practicing yin yoga on a more constant basis, where she cultivated presence and receptivity.

After a session in the Art of Co-Creative Sex program, Charlie surprised the group with this share: "I have to say, miracles do happen! Last night I had the most sensual, expanding, intimate, and pleasurable sex I have ever had with my partner. I was able to completely let go of trying to control and was able to receive and flow with his pace. It was amazing. I watched a sexy movie first and that helped…haha. But honestly, I thought this journey would take a lifetime, and it's already changed my life so much. I had a few tears of joy at the end. A true heart-to-heart connection."

She allowed herself to drop into her heart and feel. And what's more, beauty emerged from this: the possibility to fully receive her partner.

Soul Reverb

Now that you're seeing what heart-opening sex can look like, it's time for reflection. Get your workbook or journal and write down your answers.

1. If you tune into yourself, in what ways have you shielded your heart? What is your greatest fear? Can you trace back the cause of this?
2. Can you notice what gets you stuck in your head instead of feeling with your heart? In what way does being in your head allow you to be safe?

3. What happens when you drop into your heart? How does your perception change? What do you experience when your heart is present in lovemaking? What do you experience when your heart isn't present?

Chapter Affirmations:

- When I integrate my heart, it is the portal to deeper experiences.
- I am worthy to be loved fully.
- Healing my heart is what allows me to have wholehearted relationships.
- When I let the "Big Love" come in, it nourishes, enlivens, and electrifies me.

SEX ON THE CONTINUUM OF CONNECTION

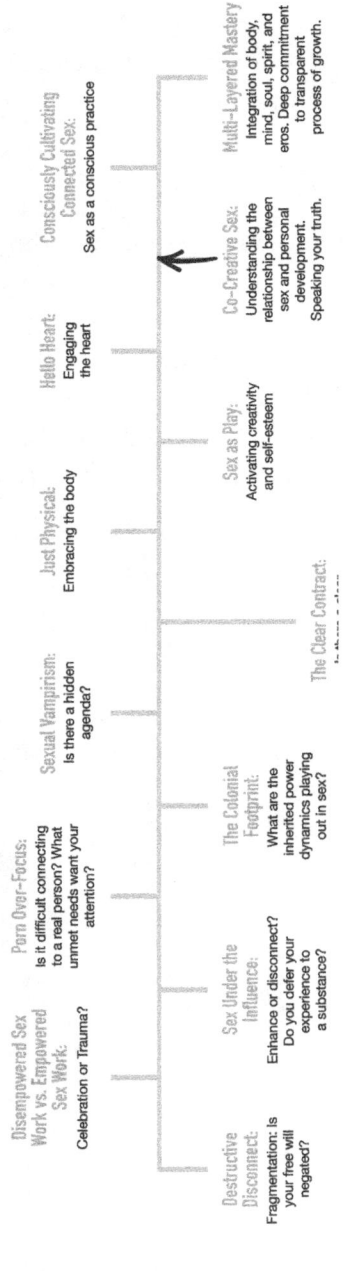

Destructive Disconnect: Fragmentation: Is your free will negated?

Disempowered Sex Work vs. Empowered Sex Work: Celebration or Trauma?

Sex Under the Influence: Enhance or disconnect? Do you defer your experience to a substance?

Porn Over-Focus: Is it difficult connecting to a real person? What unmet needs want your attention?

The Colonial Footprint: What are the inherited power dynamics playing out in sex?

Sexual Vampirism: Is there a hidden agenda?

The Clear Contract:

Just Physical: Embracing the body

Sex as Play: Activating creativity and self-esteem

Hello Heart: Engaging the heart

Co-Creative Sex: Understanding the relationship between sex and personal development. Speaking your truth.

Consciously Cultivating Connected Sex: Sex as a conscious practice

Multi-Layered Mastery: Integration of body, mind, soul, spirit, and eros. Deep commitment to transparent process of growth.

CHAPTER 10:

CO-CREATIVE SEX

"The behavior of a human being in sexual matters is often a prototype for the whole of his other modes of reaction in life."

—Sigmund Freud

When we truly become conscious agents acting in our own private process of integration, we become more whole. And when we show up whole, we attract wholeness back. The good news is that as the experience of sex deepens, health benefits do too. Research shows that our bodies enjoy a stronger immune system, reduced blood pressure, improved bladder control, and improved sleep, amongst other great stuff.[23] Sexual activity catalyzes life forces and sends them streaming through our bodies like an electrical current. These intensified life forces have the power to heal us from all kinds of past traumas and emotional blocks. They now surface and must be dealt with. With an increasing amount of consciousness, as we go up, the stakes go up. But the rewards do too.

---

23 https://www.webmd.com/sex-relationships/guide/sex-and-health#1

Co-Creative Sex

In this chapter you will:

- Discover how energy moves through your body
- Contemplate why everyone goes through the wringer, even celebrities
- See what affects us in the sexual dance
- Witness Bruno's experience with Co-Creative Sex
- Learn the core benefits and characteristics of Co-Creative Sex

How Sexual Energy Moves

Although we are taking on "Cultivating Conscious Practices of Sex" in the next chapter, I find it useful at this stage of Co-Creative Sex, to dip our toe into those bodies of knowledge that help us to better understand the mysteries of sex. When approaching sex as an art form or on a path to mastery, one has to become aware that sex is in fact a current, a life force that is impacted through breath, mindfulness, and visualization.

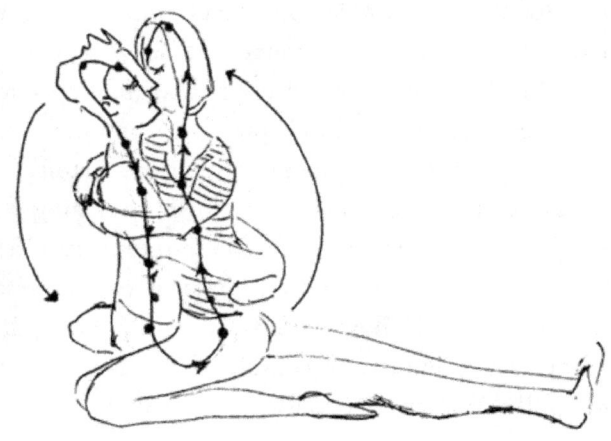

If this is surprising to you, consider this simple experiment. In *The Multi-Orgasmic Couple*, Mantak Chia and partners give an effective exercise to experience what the Taoists call chi, or life forces.

He explains that: "Usually we are not aware of this energy, which is subtle and constantly moving, but as we cultivate it, we can learn to move it with our mind and to experience its warm, tingling feeling throughout our body for greater pleasure and health." He gives his readers a challenge that you can take on now as well: Notice what happens when you focus your attention on your hands for a minute. Do you feel your hands warm up?

Western medicine is also honing in on the mind's ability to affect the body with techniques such as biofeedback, which teaches people "to control their body's seemingly unconscious processes" with their mind. Without pulling or pushing the chi, the process is altered by simply putting your focus somewhere else. Knowing that sex is this heightened life force moving through your body gives you access to a whole new dimension of possibility by learning to play with this energy. Experiencing how energy moves in your body will help you understand the principles of Co-Creative Sex.

In the tantra tradition, the sexual practice is based on learning to amplify this life force flow through the body's energy centers—called the chakras—via meditations involving color, shapes, and sound and putting these imaginations in motion up and down the central channel. I speak to you about chakras—the energy centres of the body—to better grasp the principles of energy circulation in practices such as sexual tantra.

If the idea of chakras feels abstract to you, take a moment to feel this in your body. If you've ever experienced heartache, you probably felt a certain contraction in your chest, which is in the area of the heart chakra. If there was a time in your life when you didn't feel safe, your pelvic floor probably contracted in response to fear. This is the seat of your root chakra, where information about safety is stored. And if someone humiliated you, you may have found yourself at a loss for words. You may have felt your throat constrict in response to this attack. This is the area of the throat chakra. These energy centers line up along the spinal cord, and include the root, sacral, solar plexus, heart, and throat chakras. Aligned with the pineal gland is the third-eye chakra, and the fontanelle at the top of the head is associated with the crown chakra.

As explained by Dr. Joe Dispenza in *Becoming Supernatural*, each energy center "has its own individual glands, its own unique hormones, its own chemistry, and its own individual plexus of neurons." He suggests thinking about "these individual clusters of neurological networks as mini-brains."

After a childhood of emotional insecurity, the root chakra where we store issues around security will have been impacted. If someone experiences deep heartache, their heart chakra may have constricted. Those who were bullied and mocked may have blocks in their throat chakra and may find it difficult to express themselves. By extension, the circuitry, the glands, and hormones, reorganize in a suboptimal way. As sex activates the flow of energy through these energy centers, the flow of sexual energy is arrested where there are unprocessed emotions and blocks.

The idea behind the tantra practice is to learn to dissolve these blocks to bliss, whether it be strictly via meditation or when applying it to the sexual practice itself. Because the sexual force is powerful, the flow starts dislodging some of the blocks and reawakens wounds. According to Buddhist monks, this is one of the pathways to enlightenment. In fact, orgasm is said to be fleeting moments of this high state of being.

What is useful to know regarding Co-Creative Sex is that whether or not you are working with these life forces consciously, they are indeed flowing and doing their work of making space for integration. Although you may be completely oblivious to what is activating in you during sex, you may start noticing disquieting dynamics showing up in your relationships. At this point, unconscious or inherited coping patterns kick in!

To show up for Co-Creative Sex, you must become aware that this is happening to you.

Everyone Goes Through the Wringer

No one is exempt from this process; not even our modern Hollywood gods and goddesses. These very sexy individuals appear to have it all made: beauty, success, power, wealth, and one would assume, fantastic sex! Yet when their marriages or unions erode and fall apart, we are all taken aback. We imagine that the handsome man and beautiful woman ride off into the sunset. Yet drama after drama occurs as soon as individuals start dating and having sex.

There's the Brangelina break up, the Ben Affleck and Jennifer Garner saga, or Gwyneth Paltrow and Chris Martin's conscious uncoupling. Behind bright lights are two real individuals with their own baggage, just like everyone else. Once they pull back the sheets, they too can get tripped up as those energy forces start circulating between their bodies. Why did Ben sleep with the nanny? Well … the real question is what issues were Ben and Jen not owning individually and in their marriage? Just like is often the case with the rest of us, perhaps they were ignoring the difficult conversations, or simply blind to them.

Sexual Energy, Old Patterns, and Programming

As sexual energy powerfully circulates through the body and shakes everything up, default settings kick in if they are not addressed consciously. Some people rise to meet these issues and process whatever wound or programming shows up, while many others will just continue in default mode and exacerbate the programming or the wounding, likely disintegrating the relationship in the end.

Programming comes from your own life experiences but can also come down your ancestral lineage, which the field of epigenetics is now helping us to better understand.[24] Epigenetic changes are understood as these modifications:

> "Chemical compounds that are added to single genes can regulate their activity. The epigenome comprises all of the chemical compounds that have been added to the entirety of one's DNA (genome) as a way to regulate the activity (expression) of all the genes within the genome. The chemical compounds of the epigenome are not part of the DNA sequence, but are attached to DNA. (...) Epigenetic modifications remain as cells divide and some cases can be inherited through the generations."[25]

Ancestral programming refers to emotional baggage or dynamics that were not dealt with in the previous generation and are handed down to you. In other words, you've got the hot potato now and your best choice is going to be to deal with it! Either you exacerbate it and perpetuate the cycle or decide to grow by shedding light on it, via support, coaching, energy work, being honest with yourself, naming the dynamic, speaking the truth,

---

[24] "Epigenetics has been defined and today is generally accepted as 'the study of changes in gene function that are mitotically and/or meiotically heritable and that do not entail a change in DNA sequence." Dupont C, Armant DR, Brenner CA (September 2009). "Epigenetics: definition, mechanisms and clinical perspective". Seminars in Reproductive Medicine. 27 (5): 351–57

[25] https://ghr.nlm.nih.gov/primer/howgeneswork/epigenome

taking ownership for your life, or committing to making a new conscious decision.

In the study of epigenetics, it has been found that "genes are turned on or off and can influence the production of proteins in certain cells, ensuring that only necessary proteins are produced."[26] For instance, researchers have found that "chronic exposure to a stress hormone causes modifications to DNA in the brains of mice, prompting changes in gene expression."[27]

Dr. Joe Dispenza explains in *Becoming Supernatural* that "When you change your emotions, you can change the expression of your genes (turning some on and others off) because you are sending a new chemical signal to your DNA, which can then instruct your genes to make different proteins—up-regulating or down-regulating to make all kinds of new building blocks that can change the structure and function of your body."

He goes on to explain that "if your immune system has been subject to living in the emotions of stress for too long and has certain genes activated for inflammation and disease, you can turn on new genes for growth and repair and switch off the old genes responsible for disease." With this new decision, "these epigenetically altered genes will begin to follow new instructions, making new proteins and programming the body for growth, repair, and healing. This is how you can successfully recondition your body to a new mind." As an example of this, neuroscientists have found that "gratitude literally rewires your brain".[28] They have found that levels of gratitude are linked to better moods, less fatigue and inflammation, and reducing the risk of heart failure.[29]

---

26 ibid.

27 https://www.nih.gov/news-events/nih-research-matters/stress-hormone-causes-epigenetic-changes

28 https://dailyhealthpost.com/gratitude-rewires-brain-happier/

29 https://www.choprafoundation.org/education-research/past-studies/gratitude-study/

As a culture, human beings inherit many things besides the family heirlooms. We can receive unprocessed patterns around sexual abuse, issues around racism and exclusion, tyrannical and control patterns, submissive and entitled behaviors, money and security issues, ideas around gender roles, self-esteem problems, sexist or entitled behaviors, habits of cheating, and fear to speak up. The list of insecurities, prejudices, ignorance, intolerance, and injustice can travel down from your parents, and your parents' parents, and their parents, to ultimately trip us up.

Essentially, whatever issues and emotions were left unresolved by the previous generations can be passed down to you. The only way to break the spell is to bring your consciousness to the intergenerational pattern. In fact, if you take a moment to notice, you may well discover that you attracted the perfect person to wake this up. It is comparable to two pieces of a puzzle that behave like magnets. This is what I like to call energetic correspondence; we both slide into the role we've been dealt, and it doesn't get released until one of the two becomes conscious of it and shifts out of it.

Once you awaken to the dynamic, this can allow the other person in the relationship to wake up too, but if they don't want to deal with it, then you have the first relationship crisis. When no one wants to deal with it, the two individuals find themselves acting out the default modes inherited through their ancestral and family lines.

Baljit Rayat gives very common examples of these default modes: "Jill may turn to taking care of the kids and neglect the relationship while John may turn to porn, playing video games, or watching sports." Or it could be any other distraction that suits you, like your job, working out, or social media—anything that takes up space and allows you to avoid dealing with the root problem.

And there you have it. The relationship becomes stale and disconnected. Alternately, every breakthrough, every attempt to bring clarity, transparency, and communication, brings more intimacy, depth, and connection to the relationship. It also helps to dissolve the unwanted intergenerational pattern or blind spot. Conversely, if the connection cannot be restored, it may simply shed light on the stalemate in your relationship, and you may need to confront this pattern in another way. You either dig the grave of the relationship or hit a vein of gold with unprecedented depth and satisfaction. It takes lucidity, courage, and ultimately a personal choice.

Fear will block the co-creative process. To enliven the process, you need to dissolve the fears that lead you straight into your default behaviors. Let's go back to the dance analogy I referred to in Sex as Play: if one dancer is fearful and holding back, the co-creative process is thwarted. Conversely, when standing in confidence, poise, and presence, a whole other collaboration and creation is possible. But the question remains: how do you go from fearful to confident?

Let's look at Bruno's discovery of Co-Creative Sex and how dealing with the surfacing issues re-ignited the intensity of his sexual connection with his wife.

A heads up: There may be some upsetting content in this next story.

Bruno's Story—Accessing a More Fulfilling Life

If you met Bruno, you wouldn't guess the extent of his troubled childhood. He's a vibrant and charming man with an artistic edge, whose sincerity and warmth can pull you in. Professionally, he persevered to build a successful company managing some exciting indie bands, and his success was noticed by some bigger companies who offered to buy him out. He is also the father of three children, with a charming and sincere partner.

And yet, under the surface, lots of challenges and pain plagued his life. As a child, he'd witnessed his father, who no longer lived with them, force his mother into her room. She had come out of that room in a state of shock that lasted for months. Later as an adult, he pieced together that his father had, in fact, entered their home against her will and raped her. He'd also been on the receiving end of his father's violent behavior and recalled being a small child peddling off on his tricycle, terrified. He recalls receiving handwritten letters from his dad, but this abruptly ended without clear explanation. For years he wondered why his father no longer contacted him.

Alone with his now-single mother, he had this persistent feeling that he was in the way of her happiness. He also resented that she gave away her power to abusive or manipulative men. Engulfed in her own dramas, she was not available to meet his childhood needs, and this dynamic would dig deep trenches of bitterness.

Teenagehood came with its share of torment too – drugs, porn, skipping school, and isolation. Rising conflict with his mother meant moving to a foster home. Family and home were riddled with problems and a recurring theme of abandonment.

When he met Vanessa years later, he had already fathered a child and was balancing single parenting while building up his music company. When he bumped into Vanessa in the stairwell at an event, he was completely taken aback by her. He could have sworn he had crossed paths with an angel. She was this warm, genuine, generous, and classic beauty. It seemed impossible that she would be single, and yet she was. When the two finally acknowledged their attraction, their sexual chemistry was explosive. Anywhere seemed a legitimate place to have sex; even the laundromat.

Since intense sexual activity activates pain points, the aggravated wounds from unmet childhood needs—still unresolved—would unconsciously surface. Fights and heated discussions became part of the regular relationship mix. Vanessa wanted him to come out with her friends, but Bruno couldn't stand them. They were mostly men, and he saw them as flakes dressed in phony personas. He couldn't sense anything authentic about them.

He also despised how her tyrannical boss treated her, making her work long and exhausting hours. Her boss paraded her as the sexy woman to jazz up the coordination of events. In reality, she was underpaid for hours of intense work. Vanessa always hoped for her "big break" into show business, and yet Bruno knew she was easily replaceable. In that industry, there's always a new fresh face knocking. She would come home completely spent and have a breakdown.

Her boss's mistreatment triggered Bruno, who resented how spent she was. The intensity reached such heights that after numerous discussions as a couple, he decided to take a step back from the relationship. He needed to unearth the root of this visceral reaction. After introspection and guidance, he came to understand that the dynamic was triggering his unprocessed anger around his mother. He resented how his mother gave her power to undeserving men who took advantage of her, and how Bruno bore the brunt of the corrosive dynamic in the aftermath.

By giving away their power, both his mother and Vanessa would find themselves spent and now a burden to contend with, unable to contribute to their relationship and home lives. Bruno was always the clear loser in the scenarios; again bearing the brunt of their lack of healthy boundaries and needing to pick up the fallen pieces. This was now intolerable to him.

Once Bruno recognized where the dynamic had come from, something shifted. He attended a seminar with a spiritually evolved woman, which gave him the space to process his pain and gain perspective. He then urged Vanessa to sign up as well. After they both took responsibility for their blind spots, their sexual and love connection immediately re-ignited. Whatever was in the way of the current had been removed.

Their story illustrates how personal development, consciousness, and sex are beautifully intertwined. Bruno had to process his mother's disempowerment and its impact on him. Vanessa had to learn to speak up for herself, have boundaries, and stop deferring her power to others. When you consciously trace the source of your trigger points, then clean up the unspoken suffering, the sexual connection will reflect this too.

Bruno's and Vanessa's story evolved, other issues came up, other challenges demanded stretching, their family grew with additional babies, but both continued on their path of growth, knowing the depth of feeling inherent to their relationship would surface other dynamics to process. Their job was to take responsibility for the surfacing wounds as they were made known. They also knew resources and structures were needed to support them through these moments, especially when dealing with blind spots.

In owning their surfacing shadow—their unattended suffering—they constantly replenish the fire of their relationship. It also means that their relationship becomes a form of crucible for their becoming, ignited and inflamed with sex, and the more consciously they take this on, the quicker and easier the process.

Should I Stay or Should I Go?

In Co-Creative Sex, you are responsible for your own growth. Your partner always has the choice to up-level with you or stay back in the stagnating pattern. We have free will, after all. If the partner decides to shift too, you access new levels of connection and depth in the relationship. If your partner chooses to remain in a negative pattern, then you are confronted with the question: are you committed to your own growth or do you accept to stay with your partner in this stagnating pattern? Unfortunately, the second option puts your growth on hold.

When this dynamic persists, the relationship stagnates, which means loss of vitality. Eventually, if the relationship is really off, it can become toxic—and when ignored, can lead to a painful healing crisis. Better to stay connected to your deepest truths and unwavering soul needs. Have the courage to honor them in the most conscious way possible. The surprising thing is that when you honor yourself, the world conspires to honor you too, just not necessarily in the way you were expecting. This requires you to trust and be open to receive.

Showing Up

Baljit Rayat explains in the podcast "Sex is Medicine" that in Co-Creative Sex, not only are you co-creating with your partner, but with the Universe as well, something bigger comes in to participate, supporting flow, magic, and your ultimate unfolding.

A Note for You

When you become aware of your own power and embrace being the author of your life, you realize that so much depends on how consciously you show up. You are acutely aware that the intentions you bring to your relationships significantly affect their outcome. More so, whatever unconscious fear is left unaddressed gets played out as well. This is the tricky part! Addressing them allows you to create once again from intention, from what you actually want.

When you enter sexual activity conscious of what you are bringing into the relationship, your motivations, your desires, your fears and anxieties, you also know that the sexual experience becomes an opportunity. When you ask the universe to support you, to co-create with you, help you overcome your fears, clear all your blockages, you are stepping into your self-power.

We achieve our fullest expression of self-power when we completely take responsibility for ourselves. This conscious attitude and inquiry blossoms in sexual activity. When you defer power, forfeit life accountability, and always take on the energy of others, you fall into unconscious sex where problems start taking root.

Baljit explains that when you use sexual energy consciously, all illusions eventually dissipate. You no longer believe in fairy tales, and you stop losing your precious energy. This can be, of course, a painful process when we are really attached to our illusions and we don't realize how they are depleting us. At one point, the illusions will reveal themselves, and it's not a pretty sight. Let's say you are married to someone and pretending everything is working in the relationship, when in fact, there are many unspoken issues. Just think how corrosive that is over time and what may occur! Who wants to build their life on a mirage? Only someone stuck in the middle of a desert, exhausted, and thirsty.

Furthermore, when you approach your sexual practice with consciousness, you also free your energy from being stuck in the three lower chakras. If your energy stays blocked there, eventually this may result in a healing crisis. Our life forces want to circulate; if you resist them, you are choosing its opposite: dis-ease. The healing crisis is a form of wake-up call. It's the heavy handed knock on the door.

The Maintenance Work

When you approach sex with higher levels of consciousness, you receive an extremely healing and integrative force in your life. When you tend to the process, your sexual energy will have more freedom to circulate naturally. This will catapult you to new levels of satisfaction and fulfillment, sexually and in other important aspects of your life.

So how is that addressing issues related to physical intimacy and how it can impact one's life overall?

When you process what is blocking your sexual energy, the impact reaches beyond the bedroom. For instance, if you address beliefs that severely damaged your self-esteem, and you overcome them, your self-esteem will expand and benefit all areas of your life. You may suddenly regain your self-expression, request a raise, and get it! We are active agents in the co-creations of our lives.

When consciously co-creating with sex, you become a co-creator of your own destiny. Take note: this is huge! To do this, you must address all the surfacing issues and resistances. To be a powerful co-creator, you must fully take responsibility for your life and all outcomes. In doing so your life forces become an ally, helping you access your true essence. The pain of fragmentation becomes increasingly intolerable. For instance, sex without integrating your heart, your voice, your self-worth, and even a higher sense of spiritual connection, becomes uninteresting and undesirable. Anything short of this leaves a feeling of hollowness.

The Power of Co-Creative Sex

With Co-Creative Sex, you free yourself from all your false beliefs, your wounds, your pain points, and naturally start cultivating integrity, purpose and self-realization, which leads you to authentic connection. Your life forces are always working to bring you back home to yourself, as would a strong river current. In learning to read and respond to them, you accelerate your process. This is the process of getting into alignment. Try canoeing against the current! You will experience the grueling energy-draining reality of resistance. You are resisting your own integration. You are resisting "you." When you understand the power of the current, the power of sex, you can use it for support. The conscious unfettering of your sexual energy will have a tremendous healing effect on your life. It will bring you "home" much faster!

You automatically fall out of the Co-Creative Sex process if you do things just to please your sexual partner without respecting yourself, or if you expect the other person to give you that highly sought-after orgasm. Co-creation can only happen in freedom, while expectations pull you out of the co-creative experience. Co-creation is born from the meeting of two freedoms—wanting to play and wanting to grow consciously from the experience.

The Orgasm

Baljit explains that an orgasm comes from "how energetically clear you are with yourself. And when you learn to tap into co-creative energy, you are healing all your wounds simultaneously. You are far more open, available, and entirely more connected." When individuals meet someone like-minded who "energetically" understands them, magic happens.

The crux is that it isn't how much you are energetically aligned with another person, but how energetically aligned you are to yourself. This is very powerful. Of course, when you are energetically aligned with yourself, you will be lying beside someone who is energetically aligned with you. But to attract the latter, you need to start with yourself.

Boundaries vs. Barriers

For this to happen, Baljit explains, it is very important to understand the difference between "boundaries" and "barriers." Emotional blocks and lack of consciousness create barriers to co-creative energy, whereas boundaries help you step into your power and seal against energy losses. A good boundary is equivalent to good plumbing: who wants piping to be leaking everywhere?

Healthy boundaries are made possible through healthy communication, authentic self-expression, and an understanding that honoring your needs is non-negotiable. Whereas the way you get them satisfied is entirely negotiable, the only limit to this process is your imagination and resourcefulness and receiving the stamp of approval of those involved. Imagine sex in this ever-evolving healthy container. This is the recipe for constant growth and self-realization.

The Shadow of Communication

But beware, communication can be a tool of deflection by people who are avoiding their own suffering. They may use an artifice of communication to confuse rather than clarify. This is why speaking one's truth—one's "authentic experience"—is essential. If communication is used to avoid responsibility, then we are encountering its shadow side. When people use words to control an outcome to fit their narrative, to blur the truth, or to gain power over someone, they are using the prime weapon of the sexual vampire: manipulation.

If your words are an abstract intellectual process, not informed by the heart, another shadow side of communication shows up. You'll end up focussing on unessential details that get in the way of connection—the plight of perfectionism and wanting to be "right". For authentic and real communication to happen, the heart must be engaged, and as we previously discussed, this is not easy for many people, and for good reasons! Test it out: to really speak authentically about what is going on requires courage. Find someone from whom you've been withholding and tell them what is really going on for you. Notice what activates in your heart, your throat, and anywhere else.

Your Tool for Truth

This co-creative process is an invitation to heal your capacity to speak with authenticity in real time. This skill is pivotal for Co-Creative Sex. So how can our "voice," our capacity to speak our truth, be wounded? There are many ways! Perhaps you lived in a very strict home that punished you whenever you didn't follow your parents' expectations. It feels safer to conceal the truth rather than be grounded for a week. And if you were constantly mocked for your original ideas, wouldn't you clam up as well? What if you experienced emotional abuse and were always told to just suck it up? Chances are you would come to believe your needs are not valuable and that expressing them is dangerous. Your strategy for survival involves concealing your truth.

When your voice has been disregarded, how can you communicate your needs to your partner without withdrawing or shutting down? How can you ask those difficult questions? How can you confidently express your reality? Co-Creative Sex requires that you believe your voice counts, that those scary truths are worth sharing, and that you will be heard. This is a difficult task for many people.

Courageous authentic conversations need to be practiced. If sharing your truth feels like you are jumping off a cliff, you are on the right track. You need to bring courageous conversations everywhere you go: the gym, at work, in the bedroom, in the car, at the hairdressers, in the boardroom, at the restaurant, after a long day, on your morning walk. These conversations are the energy behind your growth, and essential in renewing the co-creative energy—the very tool for connection and unleashed possibilities. It also allows you to walk around feeling empowered and self-expressed.

No need to freeze. No need to fight. No need for flight. A solid container for communication allows you to express your needs while also knowing that all have free will in the "how" of meeting the needs. This is where healthy negotiation can happen.

The Unspoken Issues

When there are unspoken issues between two people, it gets in the way of sex. Sex bears the imprint of everything that is going on. If two people are harboring anger or frustration, it is fair to say that sex will not be super connective until the resentment is cleared from the air.

Once you've tapped into co-creative power, you exude vibrancy. You become a powerful magnet for your partner and for what you aspire to. You are actively integrating your body and your sense of safety, your creativity and your sexual power, your confidence and your heart. What's more, you are becoming fully self-expressed. You also understand that the way you show up, i.e. the way you are being, has a direct impact on the outcome. If you have a habit of criticizing your partner, how else can they show up for you? Constant criticism reduces the scope of possibilities. Instead, if you figure out how to "be" in a way that invites the desired outcome, you are off to the races.

If you want your partner to show up with sensuality and tenderness, what is your way of being that will invite them into this dynamic? This is the art of co-creation here. This is a potent position to be in. As you achieve incrementally higher levels of energy, you may notice that amazing things start happening that leave you incredulous, and you realize you are co-creating with something much greater than yourself.

Your capacity to tap into Co-Creative Sex is directly correlated to your willingness to own what is surfacing—reactions, triggers, feelings—and your courage to step up and release them. Once this process is mastered, you can say goodbye to disempowered sex.

Pitfalls do happen, of course, but you'll be so much faster to catch them and rectify.

This allows you to become an empowered manifestor, creating realities that you want to experience in your leak-free vessel of love. Of course, it requires fine tuning and constant upkeep. You must stay present; there is no way around that one, but it becomes the gift that just keeps on giving, and sex will guide you there. When you are fully aligned energetically in the present, your sexual energy will nourish all areas of your life. Remember, sexual energy is a powerful creative force.

As relationships progress, your essence reveals itself one layer at a time. Your sense of safety, your creativity and juiciness, your power and confidence, your capacity to feel all need to be exercised. Here, you have become a maestro at putting your resistance aside and have refined the art of processing the "blocks" that appear.

Beyond that, you have accessed your capacity to speak your truth! Just think about it: you can express your power, your creativity, your sexuality, your boundaries, your needs, and your truth. No sexual relationship will ever be the same. Of course, communication is an art that needs constant practicing and stepping into as you grow. As you up-level, you will be invited to up your game too!

Sexual Satisfaction as a Mirror

Your sexual satisfaction is a perfect mirror of your own relationship to yourself. When you start seeing how sex mirrors your life, it will give you hints on what needs integration and access to unseen parts of yourself. When two people enter sexual intercourse from this conscious perspective, sex can yield experiences far beyond the imagined. Expand into blissfully connected sex, heightened levels of consciousness, and feelings of oneness. Above all, it reveals your true self.

On this path, you are following Isis's footsteps as she brings Osiris back to life, as she heals his fragmented state with her love and perseverance. Wholeness means having the capacity and the self-worth to receive all the good stuff you want with love, ease, and grace.

This is far from trivial. As with everything else, this happens over time. The path to becoming a fully empowered co-creator takes commitment and resolve. One step at a time. One layer at a time.

Soul Reverb

Now that you're seeing what is involved in Co-Creative Sex and what is needed for healing, it's time for reflection. Reach for your workbook or journal and write down your answers.

1. What does your "default mode" look like, meaning the behavior you unconsciously turn to as a coping mechanism? Take a moment and describe it to yourself. Do you see a pattern?
2. If issues start showing up in your relationship, how are they familiar?
3. Why is addressing this issue difficult? What is the payoff in staying attached to it?

Chapter Affirmations

- It's when I speak my truth that I allow the healing to happen.
- When I show up for myself, I allow my partners to show up for themselves. That is the foundation of a healthy co-creative relationship.
- I get to have the sex and love that simultaneously heals my heart and blows my mind.
- My way of being creates my reality and my relationship.

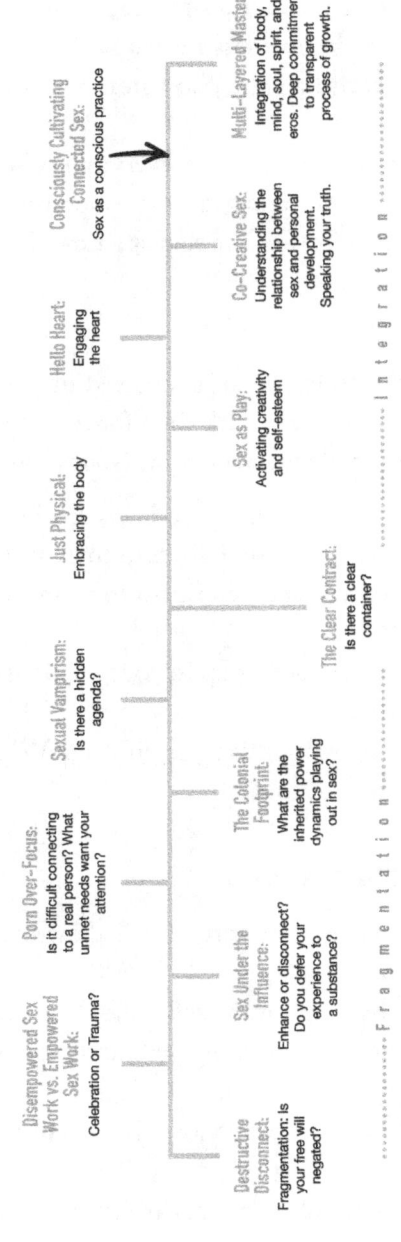

CHAPTER 11:

CONSCIOUS PRACTICES

"Sex is always about emotions. Good sex is about free emotions; bad sex is about blocked emotions."
—Deepak Chopra

We are getting to the top of the mountain and are about to stretch into the heavens. Now we can add a masterful torque to Co-Creative Sex. We have discarded the vagaries of "unconscious" sex and entered the skillful domain of striving for higher states through the portal of mindfulness and practice. This new perspective may inspire you to reconsider how you practice sex altogether.

Cultivating a conscious practice involves enhancing all areas of your sexual experience through genuine connection to self and to your partner. A variety of practices aim at achieving this goal, and I will address a few perspectives in this chapter. My first access to understanding the subtle energies at play with sex were under the guidance of Devi Ward, Tibetan tantra teacher and "Sex Is Medicine" radio host. She helped me understand the impact of connecting to self with breath, visualizations, sound, and presence. I will also share some mind-boggling discoveries experienced with

Nathan Marcuzzi's process of "de-armoring" and his "Energetic Ecstatic Experiences."

We will also take a peek into other practices such as Taoist sexuality and their "Arts of the Bedchamber," as explained by Mantak Chia and colleagues in *The Multi-Orgasmic Couple*. We will see how these various practices all seem to point to very similar experiences and appear to still evade—to a certain degree—a more Western understanding of the body. In my experience, the best way to capture this body of knowledge is in the realm of experience! Try it out. Testing things out for yourself with an open mind will lead to surprising discoveries.

In this chapter you will:

- Discover conscious sexual practices
- Try out various exercises
- Develop discernment
- Explore the Ecstatic Energy Experience
- Discover Devi Ward's story on the Power of Energy Cultivation

As we move up the Continuum of Connection, we get closer and closer to the quintessence of sex. The main goal of this chapter is to understand what can show up when you start cultivating a sexual practice in a conscious way. The study of Tibetan tantra led to life-changing discoveries for me. I learned, for one, that sex is the moving of energy between people and, when practiced consciously, takes you on a healing journey. This became clear when watching a video showcasing intimate massage.

As Devi's partner pinched, touched, grazed, and cupped her yoni, the Sanskrit word for vagina, her body jolted with electricity. Suddenly, she melted into a cathartic release. Deep sobs and tears poured out unexpectedly. As I watched, I thought *Wow. She is having an incredibly profound healing release.* Devi was releasing what she calls "blocks to bliss." Witnessing this was a revelation in my understanding of sex. Life force energy wants to circulate. We are but vessels for this flow of energy, and the less obstructed the path, the greater access you have to heightened experiences.

Tibetan tantra's secret lies in one's capacity to tap into a greater life force through meditation, then incorporate this in sexual practice. But be forewarned—as it did for Devi, this practice can involve an explosive magnitude of healing. It's a proactive way of healing your sexual *AND* spiritual energy. Through the practice of meditation and self-awareness, you learn the art of consciously co-creating using this powerful energy. As I started applying Tibetan Tantra meditations to my own practice, I experienced similar cathartic releases.

Before we deepen this perspective, I want to make sure we are on the same page about "subtle energies." To make this more concrete, let's take a moment and experience them for ourselves. You may already have had firsthand experience of them in tai-chi, qi-gong, yoga, meditation, or massage. Chinese medicine and acupuncture have mapped out pathways for these electromagnetic surges traveling throughout the body along meridians and have even harnessed them for optimal health. Western medicine has become acquainted with these subtle energies, as mentioned earlier, with biofeedback and proven how we can regulate seemingly unconscious processes of the body through simple exercises of presence, mindfulness, breathing, and focus. As explained in the previous chapter, In *The Multi-Orgasmic Couple*, the authors offer a simple and effective exercise to experience them firsthand. If you didn't try out the experiment yet, seize the opportunity now. If you did, let me give you another challenge. Focus on your genitalia instead and see if you can perceive a warm, tingly feeling there!

A Chi Exercise:

The experiment is very basic. Concentrate on your hands (or genitalia!) for a short moment. Do you notice the heat and the tingling? You did that with your mind. Taoists explain that your focus will draw the blood and the life forces—the chi—to where you put your attention. When I do it, the tingling and heat are quite immediate. Now, just imagine how you can harness this in your sexual practice, whether it be Taoist, tantra, or your own experimentation. Start choosing where you put your focus, and observe what happens to your energy.

Devi taught me how to use the Five-Elemental Meditation, an exercise in harnessing focus and mindfulness, to grow my life forces, from needle point size to encompassing multiverses, then concentrating them back into my body. Then I learned how to guide them up and down my central channel, which parallels the spine. In fact, this meditation is a form of priming of the nervous system for energy flow. Once you master this meditation, you can apply it to your sexual practice. The result: you amplify all your sensations. One reason I signed up for this program was because I couldn't figure out how to access my sexual pleasure. My sexual organs were numb. I remember wondering: Was that the orgasm? Or not? I was so confused!

In the program, I learned to give myself a yoni massage, which I remember at the time felt sort of edgy! Didn't I hear some guys making fun of women who needed to pleasure themselves because they weren't "getting any" from a man? The massage awakened life forces there, and when applying the Five-Elemental Meditation, amplified them. Through this, I initiated my own cathartic and sobbing release. As I discovered firsthand, unprocessed emotions and unhelpful beliefs do indeed block ecstatic pleasure. All those lovely, unattended feelings play hide-and-seek in our portal of pleasure.

Now that you've reached and stretched across the Sex Continuum, you may be ready to embrace a conscious practice yourself. You may already have one that you want to refine and revamp. Here are some tips to set you up for a conscious practice.

Conscious Practices for Her:

Here, the woman—or female-identifying person—no longer defers her sexual experience to her partner. Instead, she becomes an active agent in ensuring her satisfaction. She is the queen of her pleasure and upkeep of her palace. The first requirement is that she be sufficiently connected to herself to be present to what she is experiencing. With most people living highly stressful lives, the "Ocean Breath"[30] can be used to drop into your body. It's a process of re-connection and engaging mindfully with every part of your being: sexual organs, nervous and respiratory systems, heart and mind. The best place to do this exercise is in the bathtub, while the soothing effects of your breathing pulsate you up, then down in the warm water for relaxation. You are not fully in your body if you are tight and strung out. Take time to notice what can be released.

Then, put one hand on your heart and the other on your sexual organs while inhaling and exhaling rhythmically with deep, long breaths. You may realize that you've been living in your head all day or running around mindlessly. It may be difficult for you to drop into your body and connect to your heart. You have to surrender to this experience. Become aware of yourself, your feelings, and let go of anything that might be keeping you tight and contracted. Take another breath and go a little deeper.

In contrast with earlier forms of sexual disconnect, this space of self-connection is realms away from the fright of rape or from the unconscious habits of energy leakage. You obviously can't have

---

[30] Ward, Devi. (2012) Shake Your Soul Song! Dakini Dancer Press

a mindful practice if your free will has been disengaged, taken or given away. A woman's mindful presence allows her to be the captain of her own ship, the priestess of her own temple, the conjurer of her own sexual power.

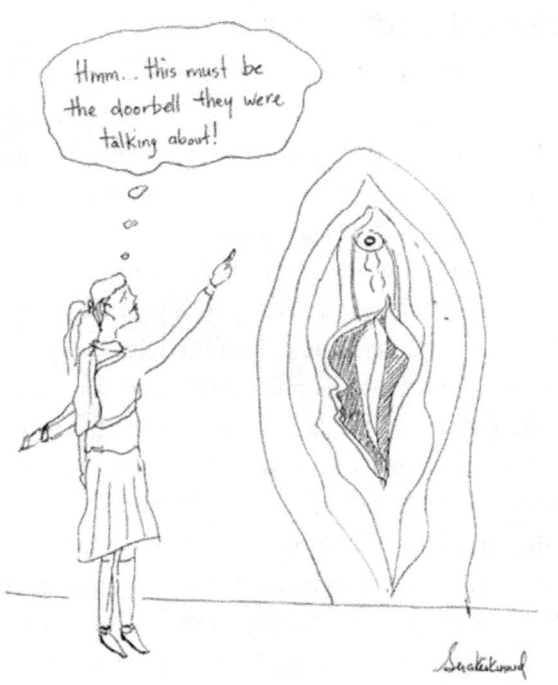

As a woman embracing conscious sexuality, the invitation is to know your own anatomy, your preferences, and familiarize yourself with your pleasure centers. This involves exploring the various erogenous zones of your body: there are twelve centers of highly sensitive tissue that can trigger orgasms for you. You can search for your G-spot, A-spot, P-spot and U-spot, amongst other zones, including the triggers in your nipples.[31] By testing things out

---

31 ibid.

through pressure, rubbing, intensity, and speed, you find how to access your pleasure. You don't need to be a master of each center, but isn't it amazing to know they exist? And finding them is a joyous happening!

Isn't it amazing to know that women's genitalia and bodies are actually designed for pleasure!? When you know yourself, you are an active agent in your pleasure and in your experience. This is another level of engagement. Just think of the tango lesson; you don't want to be falling asleep while dancing! Something happens when you take 100% responsibility for your pleasure, and it's also liberating for your partner. Of course, as a partner to women, you will also want to know more about these zones and her unique pathways to pleasure.

This knowledge and state of being is essential for women's empowerment. When you know how your body experiences pleasure, you are better equipped to guide your partner, who then has a much greater chance at succeeding in giving you pleasure. Devi always stresses this point: you can't expect another person to know innately how to bring you pleasure. You have to learn the art of communicating this and guide your partner in the most supportive way. This skillful communication increases the chances of reaching the enjoyment and pleasure you seek, and it also eliminates resentment. We are responsible for conveying our likes and dislikes, wants and needs to our partner in the most empowering way.

Conscious Practices for Him:

The man—or male-identifying person—who has adopted a conscious practice, whether it be tantra or Taoist sexuality, knows his practice depends on connecting his penis to his heart. Exercises that involve connecting breath, heart, and penis, in combination with massage, enable this. His intention is to bring pleasure to his partner. He communicates and listens to his/her needs in a safe and respectful space. He has discovered the art of the yoni and lingam massage, while also locating his partner's many pleasure centers.[32]

Furthermore, he knows, as understood by both tantra and Taoist practitioners, that his semen represents a potent solution of his life forces, which has the amazing capacity to create new life. With every ejaculation, a portion of his life forces escape him. In both these traditions of sexual mastery, the man is invited to manage his ejaculations as a means of accessing a multi-orgasmic state. At this level of presence, he comprehends that frequent ejaculation depletes his life forces, which will move him back down the continuum as he becomes depleted instead of increasingly energized and vitalized.

Semen Retention

To counter this, he develops a practice of semen retention. This means learning to orgasm without ejaculating, which—full disclosure—takes practice and commitment. Instead of being "done" after peaking once, he can sustain more sexual activity. Accessing the multi-orgasmic state involves learning to manage the intensity of arousal, training the pelvic floor muscles, weaving in breath and locating what the Chinese call the "million-dollar point" (MDP). Many men have found Mantak Chia's book and manual *The Multi-Orgasmic Man* very helpful in pursuing this Shangri-La of pleasure. You first allow for arousal, then proceed to cooling, and follow this sequence up a staircase of pleasure. As you finally peak into orgasm, you can apply pressure on the "million-dollar point" found on the perineum between testicles and anus, which enables you to by-pass ejaculation.

---

[32] Sanskrit words for female and male genitalia

In *The Multi-Orgasmic Couple*, the authors explain that by avoiding ejaculating every time, you avoid depletion: "If you have half a dozen orgasms and then ejaculate, you will lose approximately half as much energy." They also refer to one of China's most renowned ancient physicians: Sun Ssu Miao for possible ejaculation guidelines to manage their energy levels according to their age:

> A man of *twenty* can ejaculate once every four days.
> A man of *thirty* can ejaculate once every eight days.
> A man of *forty* can ejaculate once every ten days.
> A man of *fifty* can ejaculate once every twenty days.
> A man of *sixty* should not ejaculate.
> —p. 21, *The Multi-Orgasmic Couple*

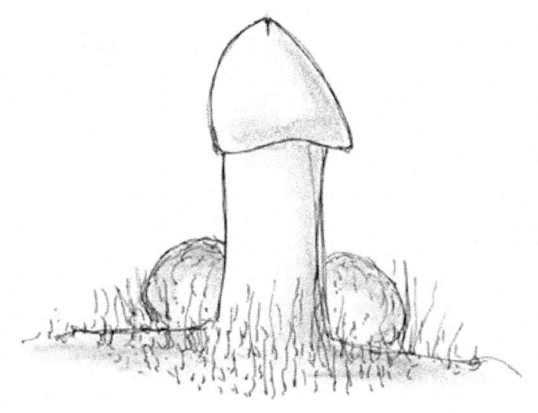

HOW TO IDENTIFY THE MAGIC MUSHROOM.

By conserving energy, the man can offer his partner a more satisfying experience too. If the partner is a woman, she often needs more time to attain higher forms of pleasure. This time may be necessary for her to simply experience an orgasm. If he can sustain, she may even access her naturally multi-orgasmic state. This means she can peak multiple times over short lapses of time. How fun to be on the receiving end of this! With the practice of semen retention, both partners can garner the benefits of multiple orgasms. Having more than one pleasure centre, a female can climax repeatedly without penetration as well. Non-binary relationships have many creative ways of allowing her to experience her multi-orgasmic state. Semen retention also prevents the disappointment that comes with premature ejaculation. It goes pretty much without saying that the practice of mutual satisfaction deepens feelings of connection and union. It can leave rapturous smiles on the faces of those involved!

The Practice

With this preparation, partners are well-equipped to achieve higher forms of connection and are encouraged to consciously connect to each other before engaging in sex. It could look like putting a hand on your partner's heart with a series of breathing exercises that allow you to fully synchronize with your partner. Maybe you deeply gaze into each other's eyes. You may breathe as you swing your bodies rhythmically together in yab-yum position, sitting with legs wrapped around each other. You may simply belly laugh in embrace. Various exercises of mindfulness are incorporated in a conscious practice of sex. Yes, you gotta drop the phone. You gotta shut off Netflix. You gotta shut the door from your family responsibilities to offer yourself and your partner this conscious creation.

In this form of sex, two people consciously want to connect through touch, breath, and gaze. They want to acknowledge the unique person in their arms and take the necessary time to do this with presence. They engage their hearts and feel the essence of their partner. Some people have trouble making eye contact during sex. It's intimidating to open up so deeply to someone's gaze, to be seen and received with such intent. Here, we are invited to garner the courage to open our vulnerable places and be seen. These are the thresholds you must cross to discover these higher places. You need to expose your naked soul to your sexual partner. Who doesn't want to be deeply acknowledged, perceived, and cared for? These qualities certainly meet universal human needs. The only thing holding us back: good ol' fear.

The Healing Properties

As you apply these practices and magnify the intensity of this energy flow, do not forget: it's pure power. These practices are designed to amplify the energy you wield, which means more possibility for cathartic healing. As you heal and dissolve your energy blocks, you increase the strength of the current streaming through your body. This current is on a mission, clearing the way to blissful states of pleasure. Yes. Here, sex become your ally.

The sex organs, the penis and vagina, become powerful tools for activating healing via the energy it awakens in the body and the processing of emotions that may occur. The penis now fully connected to the heart—becomes the all-powerful "jade stick," a healing wand, instead of a weapon at "the bottom of the barrel." The vagina becomes "the sacred space," a powerful energy center instantly felt by those who enter. In non-binary relationships, these forces play out as well. Self-pleasure shows us that we have both polarities in our own bodies. The electrical current flows on a closed circuit!

The Shadow Side of the Tantra Scene

Tantra and Taoist practices allow you to amplify the life forces going through your body, but it will amplify everything that you are, and everything that is in the way, too! If you come to your practice with poor integrity, the energy going through your body will reveal this. If you have self-worth issues, this amplified energy will shed light on it. If you are needy, your neediness will no doubt flare up. If your heart is shut down and afraid, the energy will hammer up against it until you break the armor. Whatever is shut down will be awoken and called to be reckoned with.

If you are not willing to take care of the issues coming to the surface, you are going to fall into the grips of your unconscious shadow. You will find yourself in a game of smoke and mirrors, deluding yourself. So, let's understand tantra and other practices of sacred sexuality as amplifiers and generators of growth.

This is why polyamory and monogamy—opting to be with one or more partners—are not solutions in themselves to relational and sexual bankruptcy. It is simply a context in which you discover yourself. What matters—regardless of the model of your agreement—is whether you take responsibility for yourself when things surface. Your sexual energy's ultimate commitment is to your full integration.

Maria Palumbo—"Tantra is Not Love"

Maria Polumbo is a power, sex, and relationship coach with a virtual practice that serves men and women all over the world. I was struck by one of her social media posts that went viral: "Tantra is Not Love." The title captured something I had been struggling with. Tantra is a portal to higher places, but it doesn't necessarily mean that you are an integrated person when practicing it. If you are up for the challenge, tantra will lead you to integration, but it doesn't mean you are necessarily "integrated"—nor in "integrity"—while you are practicing it. In other words, you are playing with more fire, but it doesn't mean your house is hazard free!

Fires could break out in your house, and they may be too big to deal with on your own. Learning to use tantra practices to amplify your sexual experiences simply means you know how to activate more power in the energy exchange. By extension, if your heart is shut down, you can put into action the breath work and the meditations taught in tantra, but it doesn't guarantee accessing love. In other words, if you don't know how to open your heart, you can call it tantra, and it may give you a blissful hit of energy, but it doesn't have all the possible components for connection. The experience is still only part of what you are capable of.

Maria's main complaint is that we can parade tantra as love, when in fact it can become a way of shying away from true intimacy and love. It can become a mere artifice in the art of deflecting these precious things away. She notices that people can chase the blissful, god-like ecstasy of "sacred" tantra sexuality instead of deepening intimacy with another human being. The real question she puts forward is: are you capable of true intimacy? Sex is only the tip of the iceberg. Greater intimacy comes from the sharing of yourself authentically with another person and becoming known to them.

> "I think we can get caught up in thinking breath and eye gazing and touch with presence equates a level of love. Science tells us that repeating these actions (specifically eye gazing) literally creates a sensation of falling in love over time. But something is missing. Energetic sex and orgasm that is felt in every part of the body are beautiful, but do not promise that love is present.

I think that is why there can be a deep core loneliness that is hard to quell in us who regularly practice tantra or sacred sex with many partners: tantra does not prepare us for lasting love. It creates sensation, and hunger, it wakes us up, connects us to our animal and soul. It fuels creativity and energy. But does not necessarily teach us how to be all in and let someone be all in for us.

At the end of the day sacred sex is just part of the puzzle. It is not the puzzle in itself. I think we are feeding a void with more void when we turn to sacred sex to get all of our needs met. Letting it be the solution to our desire to be radically loved.

Tantra is a way to communicate love, but it is also a smoke screen. It is a way to deepen a connection between lovers and it can also be a way to distract us. Like all good things can do."

Used with Permission From *Tantra Is Not Love* by Maria Palumbo

Maria Palumbo is a bold and courageous woman willing to express herself passionately. She stepped away from her life as a psychotherapist to pursue greater authenticity and vulnerability in her work. If she was asking her clients to be vulnerable and authentic, she felt it most congruous to model this herself. She needed to get into the court herself so she could talk from experience. Being a woman that cherishes authentic connection, she wanted to set up a conversation with me to deepen the impulse behind her article. I was delighted.

She said, "I think a lot of people in the 'sacred sexuality' community come to it out of hunger for connection, and out of idolizing sex, and I don't think they can truly fulfill their longings with the mere practice of sacred sexuality. I believe that you need to work on having a healing relationship as well outside of sex." Maria noticed that in these types of communities, depression can be a reality for a significant amount of people. "At times, it's not actually grounded in mutuality, respect, authenticity, and vulnerability. So, the sex doesn't really mean anything, it's not intimacy, it's just something really amazing. It's another quick fix to feeling good."

People engage in sex without talking about their fears, without giving space for intimacy, permission to talk about what they really want, and instead focus primarily on the sexual piece of it. "I think, as women, we get afraid to come across as being too needy, yet we want to see the man call, and so we remain unattached, but our emotional needs might not be met! We might just be giving ourselves away, instead of giving ourselves permission to ask for what we need and actually get it."

Men have the same situation. Often they don't give themselves permission to reveal and ask for what they want either. The only way to overcome fears—which could be as simple as the fear of not being enough—is by showing up for practice with authenticity and vulnerability.

The Polyamorous Lifestyle

I asked Maria about her polyamorous lifestyle and marriage. She said, "I'm not bored. I'm not hungry. I'm not needing validation. I'm not missing anything. I see polyamorous relationships as a way of creating better community, greater family. It allows me to learn things that otherwise I would never have known about myself, emotionally, physically, spiritually. It allows me to become a better person and make sure that whatever relationship it is, it is actually making my relationship with my husband stronger." She is well aware that this is not possible for everyone. "I think some people can use polyamory as a way to shift focus and lose themselves, but I use it to cultivate intimacy."

Fear of Intimacy

What Maria is looking for is growing conscious relationships in her life. "I feel like a lot of people want connection but are afraid of what that looks like; they don't want to commit and actually build relationships. In fact, often with polyamory, like with the tantra scene, there is an eagerness to have sex but not necessarily an eagerness to truly connect." She notices that she is often confronted with keeping her own desire to connect without compromising it. "Well, just having sex with this person that doesn't want to know me just leaves me unsatisfied. I mean, I try to do that, I am always walking this fine line, and I always ask myself, can I do that? Maybe in some moments it works, and in others it doesn't. I am always feeling that out."

Maria also knows that keeping your heart open is an act of courage. "Some people think that shutting down your heart to just fuck is a sign of courage, but it's actually a sign of weakness." Maria acknowledges that it takes time to get to know someone. She is also conscious that in relationships there is a lot of negotiating and expressing emotions. "Perhaps I want to feel like a priority, or perhaps when I want to talk to them, I don't want to feel like I'm always bothering them. To sort this out is basic human decency. And often I've noticed that there is so little reciprocity and little availability for healthy communication." She acknowledges that not everyone has the same capacity for emotional availability that she and her husband have.

Although Maria seems a little disappointed in how people are showing up in the tantra or polyamory scene, she also is very clear on why she wants to be part of a conscious sexual practice and have a polyamorous lifestyle. She loves her husband. He is extraordinary. "Yet there's a part of me that other people can bring out or grow or blast open because they are different people."

By adopting a polyamorous lifestyle, she says "when I finally said yes to my sex, I noticed that everything else in my life got on board. I'm not pushing. I'm not pulling. I'm just being authentic. I'm not trying to be spiritual. I'm not trying to look like a guru. I noticed that my business grew, my writing and confidence skyrocketed. As a coach, I actually want to teach people how to live with authenticity. Allowing myself to experience sex with more than one partner gave me more flavors, different energies that I had been protected against. On the other side of it, there was more energy, which meant there could be more drama, and more heartbreak too."

It's an Inner Journey

She also quickly learned that she couldn't use sex as external validation; rather, she had to learn to internally validate herself in order to find external validation. She had to learn to move past rejection. Essentially, she had to accept that rejection by someone does not decrease her worth. If her value comes from inside, she can take bigger risks, and the emotional roller coaster is minimized. Conscious relationships and sex as it plays out in polyamory is a process that is in constant flux and exploration.

Maria's main message is the importance of valuing the mundane in relationships and the importance of truly being seen, more than it is about amazing tantra experiences. "These experiences are wonderful, but they can also distract us from truly being intimate outside of sex." Are you able to be skilled, knowledgeable, heart-centered and intimate in your life and sexual relationships?

What I appreciate in Maria's share is that she is challenging everyone, even those that may be star struck with tantra or any other sexual refining practice, to always be aware of how embedded the actual intimacy factor is in the human relationship and the practice. Is it building a deeper knowledge of the other person and ultimately of yourself?

How much skin are you putting in the game? It always comes back to this: If you are following the natural flow of your sexual energy, ultimately it will bring you self-knowledge and integration. If you approach this seriously, it will lead you to a state of freedom.

Dane Tomas—"Breaking the Habit of Being Myself"

In the words of Dane Tomas, an Australian teacher for ISTA (International School of Temple Arts), a daka—the male version of tantrika—"sex wizard" and author of books *Clear Your Shit* and *Secrets from a Sex Wizard*, it's all about the big S: "Sovereignty." I've been following Dane's social media series "Dane's-Breaking-The-Habit-Of-Being-Myself-Journal." It is an amusing and authentic expression of activating and amplifying conscious sexuality and dealing responsibly with all the hidden layers that surface.

When you have a conscious sexual practice, you have to get into the habit of dealing with an accelerated rate of growth, which means developing acute vigilance. You have to get out of the habit of being yourself, consciously and regularly. It is sort of like becoming a skilled bullshit ninja! It puts you on the fast-track of true sovereignty. When we break our unconscious patterns, default modes, we are no longer shackled by them. Our actions become free, meaning released from patterns, and comes from creation and mindful action. What I enjoy about Dane's social media shares is that he always gives a quick, edgy, and authentic portrayal of where he is with his "processing" journey as he rides the waves of his sexual energy and experiences. He nonchalantly exposes his successes, his challenges, his questions, and some of his momentous conclusions, weaknesses, confusions, and breakthroughs as if they were all on the same plane of existence. To give you a taste, here is one of Dane's social media posts, used with permission:

> "Seeing lots of posts and info about open vs. closed relationships or monogamy vs. polygamy at the moment. As I go deeper into the truth of relating, conscious creation of relationship and simply practicing love, it all seems like bullshit. Actually the deeper truths are more about: Trust. The balance of security and freedom. Openness and honesty. Clear boundaries. Sovereignty. etc. The journey I perceive is about 'do I know myself and love myself enough to take care of myself.' If yes—relationships in whatever form can be fulfilling. If no—traumas will be triggered and we'll try to control things externally to compensate for the lack of safety we feel inside.
>
> And I feel internally. My inner man wants his freedom and to build his empire and live his purpose. My inner woman wants her safety, the nourishment of deep connection and to care and feel cared for.
>
> I feel more in touch with my own wounded feminine and with the crone energy than I did before. Still a work in progress, it's like we just made contact but… I can see how I've suppressed the feminine "mess" in myself and others. I can see how I've portrayed myself as 'having it all together' in various romantic connections and how actually, that's cost me love, intimacy, openness because FAKING HAVING YOUR SHIT TOGETHER creates blocks. I can see why sometimes women have given me the feedback that I'm uncaring. From the inside it's the feeling of "Oh my god I care WAAAY too much" that trips a

circuit breaker. So I run an ALOOF sort of pattern to protect my heart. It's a bit like a more sophisticated version of being in primary school and really liking a girl and going: 'Quick, she's coming! Pretend you don't like her!' LOL!"

I share his eclectic thoughts with you because this is an example of the subtext that is running in most peoples' minds, which you might relate to, and which needs to be noticed. When you are working on consciousness and sex, these are the kinds of subtle things that need to be flagged, owned and voiced authentically. To voice that subtext takes courage. It is also the perfect way of breaking the habit of being "yourself," meaning the unintentional self, the old self, the one acting out of fear, the one living out of past conclusions.

Flagging the Traps

Also to be rigorous, we need to flag some potential traps. Conscious sexuality communities are not safe havens. They are more like laboratories. This means people are playing high-stake games, getting on the court, and flirting with their edges. This also means that their shadow will surface and be invited to process it. Issues will need to be dealt with, and sometimes it will be done gracefully, and at other times, it may not. It is a constant work in progress. Let's be frank; we all have our blind spots.

Something can have the stamp of mindfulness, or consciousness, but again, illusions are easily created. Here we need to be awake and present to ourselves. To avoid any unfortunate illusions, we must address that "authority," "knowledge," and "skill" can be co-opted for power trips, games of manipulation, and taking advantage of someone's weaknesses. You can clothe the wolf in Grandma's clothes, but a wolf is still a wolf!

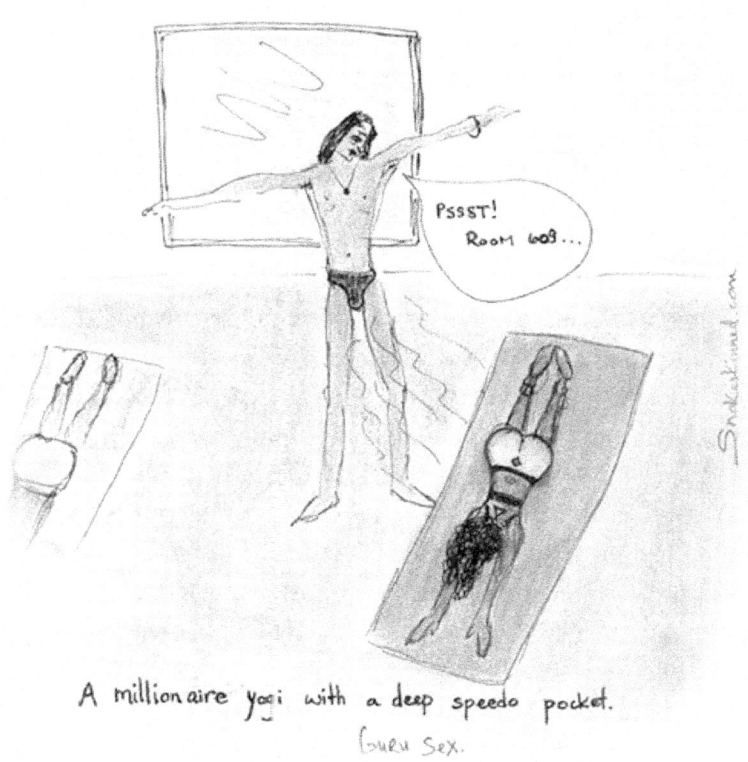

A millionaire yogi with a deep speedo pocket.
(Guru Sex.)

Abuses have been experienced in the tantra scene across the world by teachers and students alike. We are all up against the integrity challenge, and no leader is exempt. This is where you can slide down the snake's back from tantra to energy vampire.

Let's recall that to achieve higher states of sexual experiences, the containers must be clear and transparent; there can't be any energy theft or loss. We are looking for authenticity beyond the flickering lights of illusion. We are looking for a state of awakeness, authenticity, and integrity that both Maria and Dane have embraced as they consciously take on the quest of deepening connection and self-knowledge. It's a perpetual state of becoming awake and embodied. Even when you think you understand everything, something else shows up to rock the boat.

A heads up: Some content may be disturbing in the next story.

Devi Ward's Story—the Power of Energy Cultivation

If you don't pinch yourself awake from time to time, sex is going to bring a magnifying glass to anything you are avoiding about yourself and eventually bust you open. In fact, learning the art of tantra helped me understand to what degree sex can bring you to higher levels of consciousness, and if you resist, well, as they say in French: "*Gare à toi!*" which you'll come to appreciate in the next story.

As Devi Ward learned the skills inherent to tantra, her sexual power grew exponentially. She knew how to access very powerful life forces and has a remarkable capacity to channel it through her body during sex. She started noticing the necessity for her to partner only with those having a conscious practice in their life and sexuality. Otherwise, she knew her "cultivated energy" would be too strong, and she risked blasting them apart; they would simply unravel! If their shadow was too big for them to process, it wouldn't be a happy ending.

She agreed to have sex with Paul, another sex educator who practiced conscious kink. Their agreement prioritized integrity between them, and both agreed to a monogamous, transparent relationship model. Devi thought she was in good, educated hands when she started applying her tantra practice, but in reality, he could not manage the energies unleashed and this led to a meltdown. He couldn't integrate the shadow that had been awoken. The very next day he returned to his ex-girlfriend's place to have sex with her, not only severing his freshly made agreement of integrity with Devi, but also proceeded to beat his ex-girlfriend to the point where the police had to intervene and he was sent to prison for the night. He had lost both the integrity and the "conscious" in the kink.

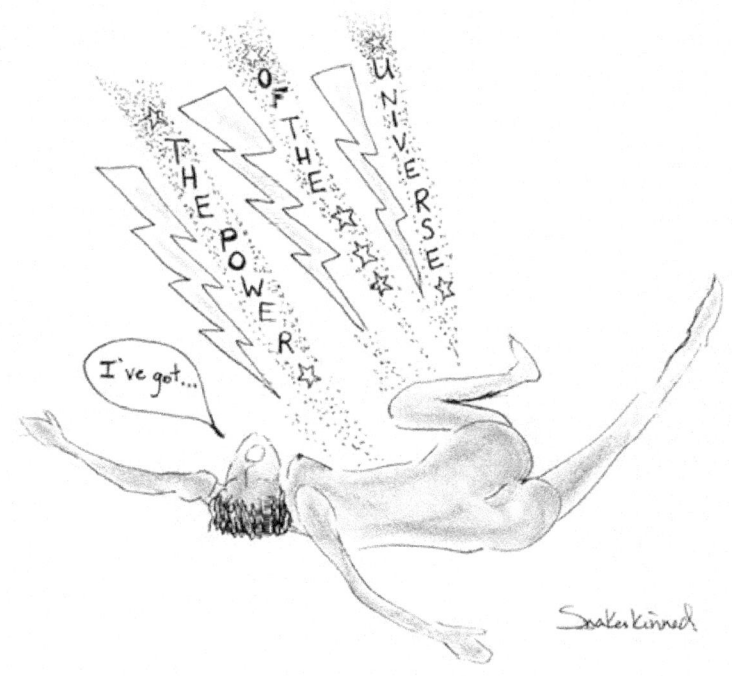

For her part, Devi's sexual experience catapulted her in the opposite direction and into a deep journey of healing, involving addressing some excruciating pain in her hip. She had to let go of disappointment, feelings of betrayal, and other surfacing issues around worthiness of being loved that she had been carrying around for the greater part of her life. In fact, this was the very thing in the way of finding an inspiring and loving life partner, what she actually yearned for.

In addressing the pain that surfaced with this event, she found herself clearing the way for her current partner, who not only deeply admires her, but is truly devoted to her as well. He is also an amazing match intellectually, on the level of consciousness, and in the mastery of the tantra sexual practice. By taking on this cathar-tic event, she had gone from a relationship of "being dominated by force" with Paul, to being "dominated by my husband's 'love', literally!" She chuckled when she recounted this. This pursuit of worthiness in love was a painful and lifelong pursuit, and it sud-denly resolved itself so gracefully after this deep purge.

The Actual Power of Sex

Devi's story is a testimony to the awesome power of sex. When you start harnessing and amplifying it, you also increase the scope of your healing experiences. When you reach this level of sexual practice, it is nothing short of a sacred and spiritual path unto itself. You have to be ready for where it wants to bring you. As Baljit Rayat wisely said, "With sex, all illusions fall."

Let the Life Forces in!

Ok, are you ready to go to an even deeper level?

When I set out to write this book, I wanted to get the bottom of sex; to go beyond everything that was ever explained to me about it and grasp what wasn't said. To understand what was hap-pening for me and for many others, and to understand why at the age of twenty I wasn't sensing any pleasure during sex when I was in love and utterly devoted to the person I was with. I wanted to understand why sex could bring people down an unfortunate spiral and completely unravel them.

And truly, this journey of knowledge has been tremendous. The number of ah-ha moments I have had when writing about sex, thinking about it, being in conversation about it, has astonished me. Every time I approached the subject something new was revealed to me. Yet, when I discovered what I'm about to share with you, I felt as if I finally found the distilled essence of sex. And it was surprisingly simple. All this time, moving life force energy through my body was so much simpler than I had thought, and it's readily available to us.

I will share with you how I discovered this. This magical experience helped me forge a bigger picture for how energy moves within us and without, which may be understood in scientific terms within a much wider scope of quantum physics. When I was eighteen and travelled to see a Mayan priestess in Guatemala, upon speaking about my parents' divorce, she took on a serious look and gazed deeply into my eyes. She said, *"Mmm, tienes dolor in tus ojos!"*—You have pain in your eyes. She then told me that if I was willing, she could help.

She led me into a small basement room with collections of relics and images. She put an egg in front of me on a small stand, lit a candle, and invoked greater forces. I am still blown away by what happened next. And as I write this, I acknowledge that it may have a supernatural feel to it, but I kid you not, this is exactly what happened—in the material world. After a few minutes, the egg in front of me literally exploded, and I started sobbing.

At the time, I couldn't explain how this had happened, but as I've become more and more acquainted with how energy can intensify in our body, and pop from the inside, I have a better sense of what took place. This was my first experience of the potential of intensifying energy through consciousness and intention. Later, I witnessed the same type of phenomena with cherished First Nations' friends. I watched them create similar types of healing spaces; as soon as the drums beats began and their voices modulated with powerful songs, the energy and emotions in the room intensified, and a cathartic healing session began. You may be wondering why I'm talking about these cathartic energy moments when this book is about sex! Let's connect the dots with Nathan's Ecstatic Energy Experience.

Nathan Marcuzzi—Ecstatic Energy Experience

One day, a well-informed friend suggested a workshop to me called "body de-armoring." Every cell of my body was a "YES!" The image of someone taking off a heavy metal armor came to mind, and the act of removing it fiercely resonated. To access the life I wanted, it was imperative that I take off my thick and stubborn armor too. It was the tough, callused armor I had placed over myself in response to what appeared to me as unchecked, unchallenged bully behavior. The only way for me to survive these stressful daily dynamics was to shield myself. But as I discovered, armors block you from the really good stuff too. It completely shuts life and love out.

So, as I lay on the floor in the dark workshop space, a workshop partner pushed on specific points: the heart, solar plexus, intercostals, jaw and inner thighs. I had previously become acquainted with the energy and emotions that tended to pool in those places, and yet I was still floored by what would happen that evening.

Nathan Marcuzzi, the humble and soft-spoken facilitator, showed us how to move energy in the body. He prefaced his demonstration by saying that he avoids calling it "tantra," as people usually get the wrong idea about it, or at least load on meaning that isn't helpful. He prefers to call it an "Energetic Ecstatic Experience," something natural and accessible to all, regardless of gender and preference. It is the art of activating and intensifying life forces and letting them flow in your body. The extent to which they appear depends on your willingness to let them in and surrender to them.

What I am about to share may appear somewhat unbelievable. The magic is in seeing and experiencing it for yourself! I want to offer you my best shot in relating it to give you access to what can happen for you too. So, I invite you to suspend your judgement a moment and be open to the possibility that this can actually happen.

Nathan sat peacefully in front of a yoga mat upon which his workshop partner lay on her back with her eyes closed. He had some tasteful, moody electronic music playing, and the lights were dimmed. The group formed a half moon around him. He began with his hands moving over her body as if he were a magician. At times he moved the air upwards from her root towards her throat, never touching, at most grazing specific points. For most of the session his hands stayed a good foot over her body. His hands would at times pump the air, and at other times he would pull a thread of air from her mouth. In full presence of his every move, he looked like a puppet master pulling invisible strings over her body.

Then, a sudden electric charge surged through her body, her toes curled, and her back arched upward. This electrical jolt ran through her, and then she fell back onto the mat. But the process continued, and the energy current grew into stronger and stronger surges. I kept thinking, *but he isn't even touching her.* Surges of energy ran through her body resembling jolts during orgasm.

Dropping Expectations

For this to happen, Nathan explained that you need to drop any expectation of outcome. The ego will block the process by wanting to "excel" or "be good at." All ego expectations need to be suspended for you to leave the head and drop into the body, where things happen naturally. I wondered if this would happen as naturally for me. I, who started off this journey so blocked, so numb. Would that volatile energy move through my body from the mere pushing of air? Was I capable of dropping into my body and letting the energy move through me?

I was matched up with a kind stranger in the room and the process began, which involved pumping the air over my body, fanning it, and circulating it up over my body, thighs to crown, without ever touching. With my eyes closed, I could sense some air blown from his mouth onto my heart. I could feel air sweeping over me. For a moment, I thought, *Well, it may not happen for me, and that is totally fine too.* But as I breathed out, some jolts started taking hold of my body. I could feel some trembles arching up my back. Through this simple sweeping of the air over my body, I was experiencing similar sensations to orgasms—waves of energy moving through my body.

Addiction to Friction

Nathan talked about our addiction to "friction," which I guess can be added to the long list of other addictions we have to getting energy hits, notably alcohol, drugs, sugar, sex, attention, and drama. When you discover how little it takes to get these sensations of heightened life forces moving through your own body, a mind shift occurs. When I sat up after my experience, I was thrilled that my body experienced the intensified energy flow. It felt like success at the end of a long journey. I had indeed let this subtle energy in, and the joy of it remained.

My workshop partner told me, "Yes, you were very open to receive!" which made me want to celebrate this momentous happening. Then, I caught Nathan from the corner of my eye. He was sitting cross-legged in lotus pose, his eyes closed, and these spontaneous waves of life forces started unleashing through him; it was the sound of a man having an orgasm, letting out a raw, male sound like he'd been punched in the stomach. He had achieved this by simply being in a state of presence and permission. This fascinated me: This experience of ecstatic energy, this orgasmic sensation, is available to us at all times. This was revolutionary to me. We contrive such complex scenarios to experience life forces and look how easy it is in reality!

I hired Nathan for a private session. I wanted to really get to the bottom of this. I had to remind myself to have no expectations and to remove any pressure on myself to perform. I had to accept just being. But mostly, I had to get out of my head. I closed my eyes. I started to breathe, and his hands started sweeping and moving the air around me. He pressed a few points: the heart, the intercostals, the inner thigh, to activate the de-armoring.

The Energetic Tsunami

Soon an emotional tsunami formed. At one moment, as I exhaled, I started to tremble. His hands continued their intuitive task. As the trembling intensified, my back arched with a mounting pressure in my heart, and emotions surfaced. Tears appeared, then sobs. His hand came to my chin, and he just held the top of my neck, putting a slight pressure on my jaw and throat.

The tears intensified, the mucus clogged up my nose, and I asked for tissue. The pain continued to spill out. All the pain I had accumulated: grief, unmet needs, disappointments, anger. I was emptying the bottom of my barrel. No need to hold onto grudges anymore! This was the culmination of all that previous work I'd done, and now, with this loosening, was opportunity. Time to let it all pour out, to purge it for good. I was ready to make room for the healthy masculine to come in, not the ailing, toxic masculine, but the wholesome and holy masculine.

I also knew all the grief, grudges, and grinding feelings were the very armor I was wearing. And I was ready to take it off. I was ready to be naked. To feel my soft and supple skin again. To feel free and ready to be loved once more; enough with this self-imposed isolation, the self-imposed asphyxiation.

And what did this do? Well, for one, the life forces in me quickened. For days after, my body felt like a pinball machine with energy bouncing from side to side, leaving a sensation of cool tingling. I noticed that I was more self-expressed. There was a glow and joy about me that caught the eye of men. I became magnetic for the masculine; men were suddenly engaging with me and appreciating my simple presence. All this happened within a few days of the de-armoring experience. Literally two days later, I began dating a fabulous man. When our sexual energy, our life force, is flowing and pulsating freely, anything is possible.

This is how I can distill this experience: The essence of sex is unfettered life forces, always available to us, moving through our bodies, and accelerating our healing.

Soul Reverb

Now it's time for reflection. Reach for your workbook or journal and jot down your answers.

1. Do you have a conscious practice around your sexuality, whether it be breathing, presencing, body embodiment practices, self-pleasure practices, tantra practices, Taoist practices, or polyamory as a form of inquiry into self-knowledge? How does this practice amplify your energy? What dynamics drain or thwart access to this energy and life force?
2. On a scale from one to ten, to what degree do you let life forces stream through your body? What is in the way?
3. Have you ever had a cathartic healing experience with sex? Describe it. What happened after? What did it give you access to?

Chapter Affirmations:

1. My consciousness determines my experience and destination.
2. The life forces are always there. I am simply the gatekeeper of the life forces.
3. My healing allows me to channel higher and higher concentrations of life forces through my body, which gives me access to pleasure and bliss—fleeting tastes of enlightenment.

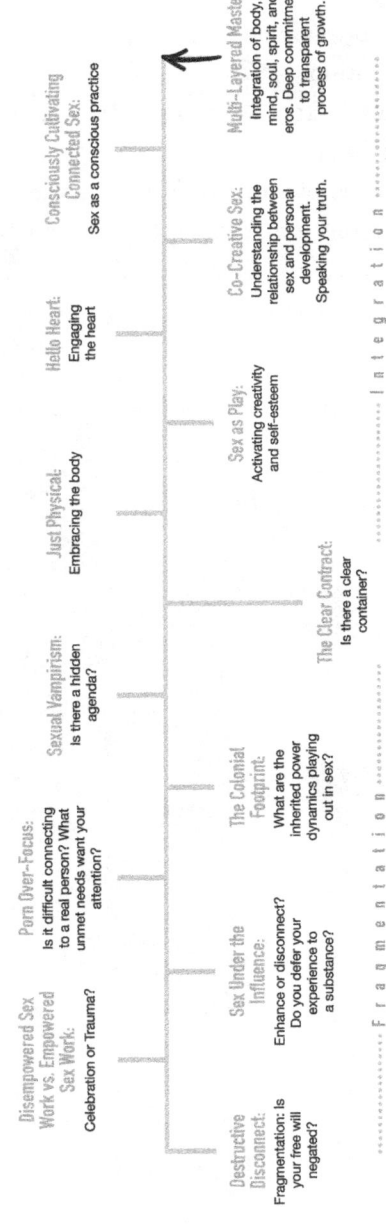

CHAPTER 12:

THE THRESHOLD OF MASTERY

"We waste time looking for the perfect lover instead of creating the perfect love."

—Tom Robbins

What a journey we have had. From destructive disconnect to blissful sexual connection. Throughout this journey, the common thread has been, the process of becoming more and more conscious of what is happening to our sexual energy and owning it. Being authentic about it. Voicing it. And taking care of it. The more we clear our inner emotional blocks, the more we experience our true essence and the more we reach higher-frequency relationships and sex. They go hand in hand. So, here is the last stop on the Sex Continuum. We are reaching the big "O," not so much as in orgasm, as we typically think of it, but as in becoming the "One."

When Eros, love and sexuality finally fuse together, you are traveling the path of self-discovery. Love seeks more depth as your energy uncovers what needs healing. It allows you to rebuild yourself to wholeness. Here you are on the path of deep transformation; it is the alchemy of your soul.

The Threshold of Mastery

In this chapter, you will:

- Understand what happens when you integrate sex, body, heart, mind, soul, and spirit
- Discover a roadmap for creating a new model of spiri-tual commitment
- Experience Destin Gerek and Elie Prana's story of being on the threshold of multi-layered mastery
- Identify what you really need to cultivate and fully embrace high-voltage connective sex

If you remain deeply committed to this path of self-discovery and growth, your connection and development can take leaps and bounds. Your intimacy, your being "known," keeps growing beyond the physical, emotional, and intellectual. You deeply connect on a spiritual level as well. This is the place where sex, body, heart, mind, soul, and spirit become whole. And you may now be wondering how you can sustain that over longer periods of time!

When you've achieved a connection on all these levels, it produces a feeling of ultimate connection: union. Such levels of transcendence with another person gives you a feeling of coming "home." This may inspire you to want to commit to this person at a whole new level. Here, a new model of marriage is possible: a marriage that requires new levels of inner commitment, mutuality, and consciousness.

Before we go deeper into this new model of commitment and what it requires, I would like to address some concerns. Many people associate marriage or long-term commitment to a death sentence for attraction and sex life. In *Mating in Captivity*, Esther Perel talks about the paradox between an increasing intimacy and a plunging sex drive: "Love seeks closeness, but desire needs distance." And this we all know to be true: we've all heard about sexless marriages, we've all heard about people losing their libido in relationships overtime, and perhaps have even experienced it ourselves or been a witness to it up close.

Long-term-ness

And yet, we have all spotted at least one phenomenal couple that seems to sustain love, passion, and sex over long stretches of time, and we wonder: *How do they do that!?* For one, Mantak Chia & Co present a very different view of "long-termness" in *The Multi-Orgasmic Couple* that comes from a three-thousand-year-old tradition of sexuality:

"According to the Taoists, it takes years to reach the heights of physical, emotional, and spiritual union. It was often said that it takes seven years to know your partner's body, seven years to know your partner's mind, and seven years to know your partner's spirit. According to the Tao, it takes twenty-one years just to get acquainted! The longer we are together the more we know each other and the better our bond."

Chia and company also refer to Robert W. Levenson's study from the University of Berkeley that suggests that, in contrast to popular belief, "What we actually thought we would see is a kind of fatigue quality in these (long-term) relationships. But that's not what we see. They're vibrant, they're alive, they're emotional, they're fun, they're sexy, they're not burned out."[33] And according to another study, sexually active seniors are amongst the happiest!

So, what produces such different results for couples? Why do some couples go down the path of boredom and loss of libido while others manage to sustain and cultivate sexual connection? And if we take this to another level, how does union continue to yield a continuously deepening and satisfying sexual connection?

---

33 As reported in the Los Angeles Times, June 4, 1995.

What I've noticed is that the more we become conscious individuals, the more we are invited to create our lives from intention. The more we step into being the creators of our lives, the more we must generate the desired, co-created outcomes from our own determination—from a place of freedom and sovereignty. The same is true for relationships and sexual aliveness. As relationships progress, there are many opportunities that present themselves.

I often think of it as a board game of Snakes and Ladders. Some situations invite us down the slimy backs of snakes into lesser connection, at times sterile disconnect, and other situations allow us to rapidly ascend the ladder to new heights of vivid aliveness. And there are various qualities and ways of being that allow for such things to occur and determine the outcome.

The Transparent Process

In her book *Creating Union*, Eva Pierrakos gives a useful road map to achieve these types of unions, in constant ascension towards lofty experiences, aliveness, and profound connection. It involves a new form of transparence which, when practiced consistently, generate a whole new possibility for long-term commitment and marriage.

> "The new marriage is totally open and transparent. There are no secrets whatever. The soul-processes of the partners are totally shared. This openness and transparency has to be learned. It is a path within a path, as it were. Expose your difficulty in achieving this openness, rather than trying to deny or hide it.
>
> Part of the openness consists in revealing your fear of the strong spiritual current, of the forces released by the unification of your sexuality and your heart. When the fear is shared—even though you may be

unable to shed it as yet—the obstructions will be eliminated relatively fast, and a kind of vibrant fulfillment will come from the sharing itself.

(…) Being on a path of profound self-development and shedding light on the hidden parts of the self are prerequisites to fulfillment in an alive and vibrant relationship. When the vibrancy ebbs away, the causes need to be explored by both partners together. There may be any number of reasons for the stagnation, none of them necessarily bad or shameful. (…)

When all levels of the two personalities are open to each other, join, and finally fuse, the intensity and vibrancy of the sexual encounter will surpass anything you can at present imagine. This kind of fusion cannot come about easily. The fusion on all levels of the personality means the fusion of all energy bodies. This is rarely the case. You will come to know when the fusion exists only on the physical level, and when it happens on the emotional, mental, and spiritual levels. (…)

Bliss, ecstasy, pleasure supreme can never exist gratuitously, can never be cheaply snatched. They could not be born that way. They can be born only when the personality has reached sufficient purification, security, faith, self-knowledge, comprehension of the universe."

Pierrakos talks about some very important elements for this level of connection to be possible that I'll sum up as:

1. Radical authenticity
2. Vulnerable self-expression

The Threshold of Mastery

3. Active flagging, owning, and sharing the surfacing fears
4. Being 100 percent responsible of self and the created relationship

In one of her social media posts, Layla Martin, a well-loved sex educator and tantrika, explains how her partner of many years and herself are still unearthing dynamics that can get in the way of love and how their renewed commitment to growth allows for sustaining relationship abundance. Here, she explains why relationships require work and what that looks like:

"Relationships are hard work because they are reflective mirrors that bring up all of your issues around self-love, intimacy, self-worth, sexuality and everything you wish you'd gotten from your parents but didn't. The relationship is an invitation to heal yourself on all of those levels so that you can love and see each other clearly. It requires healing and integration of mind/body/soul levels and if you don't do it, you'll fall out of love and stop having sex."

She then explains in more detail what the "work" entails. "Understanding your own triggers, projections, stories and wounding patterns and engaging with a healing process that allows you and your partner to hold them compassionately and for you to integrate them back into wholeness."

Bingo.

The best part is yet to come. "Why is it hard? Because most of us are taught to run away from our wounding and fears: to hide, lie, avoid, deny and deflect. So the most natural approach is to blame your partner, your relationship and/or yourself rather than fully open up to and explore your vulnerabilities and take full responsibility for the relationship your create."

Layla also distinguishes between working at something and simply hanging on out of duty. "Also to keep your relationship alive you have to sacrifice it every day, which is scary. You have to have a higher value of love, truth and aliveness than just hanging on because you're supposed to. It takes real courage to choose that every day."

To find this level of connection and long-term commitment in the "real" world is not an easy shoe to fit. An enlivened relationship, erotically charged, ensouled with deep love and commitment that perseveres over time requires masterful people.

For one, traversing a sufficient number of important trials and demonstrating a sincere and authentic level of commitment, which does not limit this type of commitment to a closed-relationship or monogamy, but means that all agreements in this union are born from transparency, free will, and communication. Another is being able to successfully upgrade one's intimate connection, overcoming challenges in the relationship multiple times, getting through the eye of the needle, or through the crucible of purification, coming out of this process transformed, empowered, and awakened.

Finding a couple that has been sufficiently prepared and empowered to fully reveal every single aspect of their soul life, desires, and impulses to each other, requires some sleuthing! Finally, it demands that both partners show up for their respective partner as much as showing up for themselves.

Thankfully, all my sleuthing has produced results. I met Destin Gerek through my interview process and spent hours listening to his edgy and fascinating sexual biography.

Destin Gerek and Elie Prana's Story— Multilayered Mastery

I met Destin Gerek when I started researching and tackling the very broad topic of sex. I was listening to collections of "Sex is Medicine" podcasts and was attracted to one called "The Demonization of Male Sexuality." Curious, I listened and was impressed with the sensitivity I heard in Destin's voice. He did not opt for the Pick-Up Artist (PUA) routine of manipulative and deceitful tactics to break through a women's defenses for sex. Instead he explained how men can create a truly safe container for women that actually ignites their passions and desire for sex rather than force it on them.

Destin was not impressed by the pick-up artist mentality and instead sought to attune to a woman's experience, responding to her every expansion and contraction, making her feel inherently perceived and safe, so that she unleashes her sexual power out of her own volition when she is ready to do so. There is no need for pressure or coercion here. He promoted the possibility for women to feel entirely safe, respected, and turned on simultaneously.

For that time, this was a definite leap in consciousness. This was not the common "locker room" bragging being shared amongst men. He believed there was something beyond being that "self-centered-bad-boy-asshole" who is simply taking what he wants from women, or conversely, the asexual "friend-zoned" man who lost his balls. One could take the best of both worlds, the passion and the animalistic desire connected to the heart.

Who was this man caring so much about women and their sexual experiences? I was impressed and wanted to understand how he had come to such empathetic insights. I was a little intimidated by what I discovered on his website. His chiseled and tanned chest tattooed with a huge mandela covered the screen. He definitely exuded an erotic masculine power. Funnily enough, I felt too intimidated to reach out to him because of it. *Usually these kinds of guys are so full of themselves*, I thought.

But nonetheless I started following his Facebook page. And a few months later, he wrote a sincere post that really struck me as coming from a deeply lucid and heart-centered place. He was addressing some illusions in his life and was authentically sharing about them. *This guy has substance and depth*, I thought. *I have to speak to him.*

I reached out to him and he kindly accepted my invitation to share his story from his sunny Californian home. I wanted to know how he had become so committed to upping consciousness around sex and sexual dynamics. What I discovered was instructive. He hadn't always felt erotically empowered as a man. In fact, for a large part of his teens and up until his late twenties, he was very angry with everything that was masculine.

He grew up in a dysfunctional home of pent-up frustrations. His mother, a morbidly obese women whom he dearly loved, was his protector. She was also a source of deep embarrassment, as he faced the teasing and bullying from other boys in his neighborhood. His father, although mostly absent, would overflow with resentment and frustrations towards his wife when he was home, compounding Destin's mother's low self-esteem. Destin experienced many scenes of verbal denigration, which he sometimes bore the brunt of as well. It would only be years later on his healing journey that he would better understand the dynamics at play and his father's deep feelings of disempowerment.

In addition to this, he discovered that his high-school sweetheart had been raped on her fifteenth birthday by her previous boyfriend. It turned out that Destin was the first person she confided in and he was besieged by an overwhelming anger. Flashes would overcome him where he would be "throwing this unnamed invisible boy against the wall and hammering nails into his testicles one by one." He spent countless nights holding his sweetheart's hand in the bathroom because of the excruciating pain of her many urinary tract infections. Later, in college, many women confided their experience of some form of sexual assault or sexual coercion. It appeared to him that the world was in the throes of an ongoing sexual assault epidemic. He recalls making a vow to the Universe, saying, "I am committing to create a future in which we look back to sexual assault as a mere relic of our more barbaric past."

The Threshold of Mastery

For over ten years, everything "male" seemed wrong and would be canceled out of his life. He believed men were dangerous, especially their sexuality, until he started noticing how out of balance his life had become because of this belief. He had, to a certain degree, dissociated from his masculinity. The drawbacks showed up in his relationship with a woman he truly loved.

He had put her on a lofty pedestal, amazed by her powerful and sexy creative spirit. Whenever there were issues in their relationship, he always thought it was because of him. Yet, angry with his meekness, she not only asked but demanded that he step into his masculine. Destin realized he didn't know how to do that. His partner's rage ignited his intense journey to find his masculine and become the male role model he would have wanted for himself.

He created an alter ego, the "erotic rock star." He would wear this persona before going out or attending festivals, and to his great surprise, it allowed him to tap into a sense of power he didn't know he had. This persona was attractive to women; it worked beyond his wildest imaginations and brought new energy to his relationship, even if it subsequently ended. Regardless, he felt infinitely grateful to his partner for inviting him into the intense, purifying crucible that allowed him to embody his manhood.

As Destin says, it allowed him to discover that, as a man:

> "You can embrace your sexual power. You can have plenty of lovers and whatever degree of casual sex you want AND you can do so without leaving a wreckage behind you. Men tend to follow one of two paths. Either they just follow their sexual desires without care or attention to the impact they are having or they are so afraid of being that they cage their masculinity and disconnect from their inner power, sexual desires and expression. They want to be good men. But instead, they become nice guys. People-pleasers. Not

in touch with their true desires because they are so concerned with getting approval. External validation. They lose touch with their inherent power, because they are afraid of it. And because they feel they don't deserve it."

He saw another route than the upheld idea of "I should meet my needs at your expense," and that it was possible to have your power co-exist aside someone else's. It wasn't an "either/or" situation. These ideas would become foundational to the creation of his "Evolved Masculine" movement, where he is challenging an army of men to stand into their masculine power while standing up for the respect of the feminine, which one can witness in the likes of Michael Ellsberg's pledge to gather 10,000 signatures of men committing to sexual consent. Destin Gerek's vision and commitment to the Universe as a young adult is taking root in the world.

After six or seven years with the Erotic Rockstar, Destin felt he had gotten what he had needed from it. He noticed that his desires and what he wanted in life had changed; that he had indeed graduated from the persona.

From the start, Destin's biography intertwined the theme of sorting through sexual issues for himself, alongside supporting others on their healing journeys, whether it be as a lover, as a certified sexological bodyworker or as a trained daka—a male practitioner of tantric yoga. And every step of the way, he was willing to rise above cultural conventions and challenging taboos to fully embrace his deep truths and meet the true soul of sex in freedom. This process involved healing his own family baggage, setting boundaries, embracing his sensitivities, and growing his emotional discernment. It also meant finding a new paradigm for embodying his masculine sexuality and stepping into the world with it.

The Threshold of Mastery

While most of his committed relationships throughout his life involved a deep level of love, and an enviable level of sexual chemistry, they were always intertwined with high levels of drama and at times, toxicity that eventually would erode them. A common pattern that he encountered was that all of his partners had experienced sexual trauma at some point in their life, which no doubt increased the stakes for conflicts and issues to disentangle.

Over the years, his desire to reveal sexuality at its fullest expression while holding the highest esteem for integrity was a deepening path with many heartaches. But the beauty of his process of growth is that it led him to the woman with whom he would decide to take one step further with a formal commitment.

Elie Prana entered his life as a member of his circle of friends, witnessing his various tumultuous relationships, then eventually as a lover. Elie Prana's manner sharply contrasted with the high drama he'd been accustomed to. It was almost disconcerting to him: love and passion had always meant drama in the past. Now, there was always room to address their problems within a safe container. Destin noticed how different this made him feel, and this was increasingly cherished by him. It was time for him to shed unnecessary drama from his life, something he had lived with since childhood.

Their relationship evolved over a long maturation of ten years in which they had grown to know each other deeply and authentically. It also meant that regardless of any discord that would emerge, they knew the relationship was a perfectly safe container for both of them. One day, Elie Prana challenged Destin: "Why do you always choose wounded women?" This required some deep reflection on Destin's part. He did recognize the pattern. Looking into some of his own family dynamics helped him understand that he had become, in some ways, the emotional caretaker for women in pain.

Elie Prana had experienced sexual trauma also, and its pain started surfacing as their relationship deepened. She had to process the abuse of a "destructive discipleship" with a guru. Elie had decided to break away when it became clear that it no longer supported her heart's deepest desire: to be with Destin, the man she loved.

In this discipleship she submitted her ego as a path to enlightenment leading to abusive power dynamics and sexual abuse. When Destin re-entered her life, the toxic dynamics in this discipleship were apparent to her, which made her want to renounce this spiritual path. She felt lost and confused, with an eroded sense of identity. Destin suggested she try a sexual healing program called "Pleasure on Purpose" with Jonathan and Heike. Within this context, her troubled emotions of the physical violence of her childhood and teenage years surfaced and were addressed for the first time in a very tangible way.

She was trying to break up with a boyfriend at age nineteen, when he locked the car, covered her mouth, and raped her. When she finally managed to scream, he told her, "No one is going to hear you." He then photographed her and threatened to post the photos online if she dared speaking. When Elie had finished her healing process, she encouraged Destin to consult with her mentors as well.

Destin was inspired by her transformation and how she had reclaimed her voice and her power. She was fearless, having worked on almost all the wounds of her past, and it became clear that it was time for him to "clean his side of the street" too. Regardless of all the transformational work he had done throughout his life, there was still more to process. His sessions helped him purge blocks he did not even know he was carrying.

Elie stated that it was beautiful to experience as a couple. Going through this profound experience of energy clearing was one of the best decisions they have made. They did the inner work on their own and came together with an even greater heart capacity. They credit their ever-deepening bond to this healing experience. I must say that the quality of their communication and courage for authenticity is what keeps and renews their bond. I interviewed them separately, and I was moved by how much consideration they have for each other. They made it a priority to always check in and make sure they both had a voice in the direction they had adopted.

A few months after our interview process, I found out they had gotten married. All their respective work cleared the way to wanting to take a step further and fully commit to each other. Together they have chosen to cultivate love, passion, pleasure, erotic exploration, and mastery. They are committed to integrating all layers of their being within their created container of consciousness. No matter what trigger points get pressed, there is a commitment to show up, share, and transform to cultivate aliveness. This story is a powerful expression of inner work, speaking truth vulnerably, and being 100% responsible for your life, and your sexual practice, as you progress towards multi-layered mastery and integration.

Here the sexual connection works on all levels, fusing Eros, love, and sexuality with body, soul, and spirit. The key word here is "intentionality."

Are You Ready for High-Voltage Connected Sex?

As described by Pierrakos, when the deep-seated fears are addressed, when authenticity reigns, when the sexual stream is awakened and cultivated, when sufficient purification has been achieved, the result is high-voltage connected sex. As mentioned in the path of Taoist sexuality, commitment to "knowing" body, mind, and soul takes *time*—twenty-one years, they say! The looming risk, as highlighted by Perel, is death by proximity. The antidote is really taking on intentionality and creating the conditions for success, searching, and generating them. Be astute, awake, and calibrate when things fall out of alignment. It's being 100% responsible for all your experiences.

As mentioned in earlier chapters, high-voltage sex dissolves all illusions. Bliss without building an intimate, mature, and masterful container will cause relationships to fall apart. In a blissful connection at this stage, it is important to know that if you are not prepared for such high-voltage energy during sex, the high-energy currents will simply melt you down. It's sort of like an overdose: the energy is too powerful for you to deal with, as we witnessed in Devi's story with Paul.

Those who reach states of enlightenment have achieved it through a long process of purification. Sometimes people choose to experience high levels of pain before shifting or shedding, before accepting to see the illusions they operate in. Sometimes our attachment to illusions can be strong. Letting go can feel like death.

If you have found your way here, you have tasted the elixir of enlightened relationships, and perhaps enlightenment itself. You are given access to blissful oneness. You have fused many parts of your being back into a whole: sex, body, heart, mind, soul, and spirit are now fully working together as a team. When sexual practice involves such levels of intentionality, fragmentation melts away.

Everything leans towards the all-encompassing One. You. Your partner. The Universe. And Beyond.

Soul Reverb

Now that you're seeing what is needed for healing, it's time for reflection. Reach for your workbook or journal and write down your answers.

1. Are you scared of commitment in a relationship? Be honest, what actually scares you? What is underneath that fear? Where does that fear come from?
2. In what ways are you scared of committing to yourself? Why?
3. In what areas of your life can you become even more transparent? In what areas of your life do you need to amp up your courage so you can be fully "known"?

Chapter Affirmations

- When I speak my truth, I honor my soul.
- When I honor my soul, I can show up for myself and for someone else.
- When I commit, I am allowing myself to be known and delight in this intimacy

The Higher Continuum: Fusing into "One"

This is the journey. From destructive disconnection to multi-layered mastery. We started with violation and sexual assault, and the fragmenting of our basic human life pulse: free will. Then we discovered the various ways a sex worker can show up, whether it be from an empowered or disempowered place, and how that determines the outcome of the experience. Is it a celebration of sexuality or a re-traumatizing based on past events? Then we looked at sex under the influence to determine at what point you defer your power to the substance, if at all.

We explored pornography and porn over-focus and some of the unmet needs that are being expressed when stuck in this over-consumption. We looked into sex and the colonial footprint and what it involves to actually decolonize and "free yourself of mental slavery." We explored how shame has got to go then moved into the greyest zone of the continuum: the covert qualities of sexual vampirism and uncovering hidden agendas that may play out.

We saw that when coming from these places, sex has a fragmenting quality. It erodes, breaks, and blasts delicate parts of your being into alienated pieces. One shard of genitalia may be broken off and a piece of heart may be stranded and adrift, and the two shall never meet!

The journey, as I discovered myself, is about traveling from fragmentation to integration. It's the exact path Queen Isis followed as she collected the scattered pieces of her beloved Osiris and fused them back into wholeness, into the full integrity of his being, piecing back together arm, leg, heart, belly, head, finger, thumb. It was the love in her heart that mended the fragmented pieces of his body back together—minus the final limb. In my opinion, the best way to access the wisdom of mythologies and fairy tales is to look at all the characters as representing a facet of ourselves. We are both Isis and Osiris on this journey of fragmentation and integration. And if we are willing to go one step further, we are Set as well! As we saw with these collected stories of struggles and breakthroughs in this book, the Egyptian myth illustrates the very process we must undergo to heal ourselves: journey to gather all those scattered pieces and bring them back into a whole.

This involves inhabiting the body, releasing shame, freeing creativity, reclaiming power, unshielding the heart, unfurling the voice, unmuting the inner voice, and learning to give weight to intuition and discernment as you co-create your future becoming. These are all the elements that, when re-integrated back into wholeness, allow you to finally become "Your Highness." You've become a sovereign being, a place of powerful creation. And since sex is a creative act, let me tell you, you will be going places! Sex, body, heart, mind, soul, and spirit are now working as a full-on

The Threshold of Mastery

power team. When you achieve this, you will experience a glimpse of "The Great Peace." Like my wise massage therapist loves telling me after each session: "Welcome home." Until then, remember it's a process, and you always deserve kindness. Treat yourself with a lot of self-compassion and indulge yourself in the very loving of your own being.

Congratulations on your courageous journey of integration. Coming out of this journey together, with the many discussions and angles explored in this book, you should have a better understanding of all the parts of life that impact your sex, and how sex impacts all the parts of your life. Now go and live your best sexual life! Sex UP your life, UP the Continuum as you tread your unique path to integration!

ACCELERATED HEALING

An Invite!
As I worked through all this material and removed blockages on my own path, I came to see some of the archetypal issues that fragment us. I also witnessed how we can accelerate the integration process through the help of the Akashic Records and by accessing the infinite field of possibilities. By creating a sacred vessel for healing, you can jump ahead.

As I deepened my process in conjunction with working with clients, programs to heal sexual energy emerged. They are designed to allow you to show up differently both in sex and in your own life, as everything is so beautifully connected. My commitment is in helping you become whole.

To learn more about this, go to www.cocreativesex.com and we will find the right program for you.

Let's get the process of integration happening for you! Your sexual energy is an integral part of who you are, and in the process, we will be actively integrating all the other layers that make you fully "YOU." Just imagine who you'll be once all those broken pieces are brought back into wholeness. Image the depth and satisfaction of the relationships in your life.

Revolutionary.

You won't recognize yourself.

Talk to you soon.

ABOUT THE AUTHOR

JULIE ARCHAMBAULT is a holistic teacher and storyteller for all ages using pedagogical stories, archetypal mythologies/characters, collected stories, along with personal ones to inspire readers, students, and crowds alike.

Creativity being a guiding principle in her life, Julie is always searching for ways to innovate our social realities. Whether it be for the well-being of children, teenagers, or adults, she takes a stand for a holistic understanding of human development and self-realization.

The founder of CoCreativeSex—a wellness business committed to powerful lives, powerful relationships, and powerful sex—Julie forges a new paradigm where sex, relationships, and personal growth go hand in hand. By teaching her clients how to heal their sexual energy, weed out the toxic programming, and embody their fullest human potential, she creates opportunities for her clients to step up in their relationships, their sexuality, and all areas of their lives.

She works both with private clients and groups via one-on-one coaching and online/live workshops on the themes of sexuality, creativity, power, and courageous conversations.

Julie has made Vancouver, its coastlines, and sunsets her place of happy dwelling.

HELPFUL LINKS

SEX UP YOUR LIFE WORKBOOK:
cocreativesex.com/workbook

Resources:

Devi Ward: *Authentic Tantra*
authentictantra.com
Sex is Medicine,
tunein.com/podcasts/Health-Home--Life/
Sex-is-Medicine-with-Devi-Ward-p731898

Destin Gerek: *The Evolved Masculine—Claim your masculine power, become an evolved lover, and create the life of your dreams.*
fb.com/destingerek
fb.com/evolvedmasculine
twitter.com/destingerek
instagram.com/destingerek
youtube.com/user/destingerek

Helpful Links

Hasina Juma: *Empowering Bisexual People of Color and Their Families*
Hasinajuma.com

Dane Tomas: *Sexuality, Magick, Consciousness, and Business*
Danetomas.com

Diane Hill: *Ka'nikonhriyohtshera: Fostering the Emergence of the Good Mind—An experience in Quantum Energy Integration*
Dianehill.net

Layla Martin: *Epic Sex and Legendary Love*
Laylamartin.com/
instagram.com/thelaylamartin/

Seani Love: *Conscious Kink, Shadow Tantra, and Journeys into the Sacred Mysteries*
seanilove.com
schooloferoticmysteries.com

Maria Palombo: *Fall in Love With Yourself and Get Unstoppable*
mariapalumbo.com
facebook.com/maria.palumbo.loves

Baljit Rayat: *Akashic Soul Readings and Star Activation Soul Blueprints*
lotusdestiny.com
facebook.com/lotusdestiny/
instagram.com/lotusdestiny/
twitter.com/BaljitRayat

Nathan Marcuzzi: *Body De-Armoring and Energetic Ecstatic Experience*
dearmour.me/

Julie Archambault: *Healing Coach, Sacred Container, Akashic Soul Readings, The Art of Co-Creative Sex Online Healing Program*
CoCreativeSex.Com
instagram.com/cocreativesex/
facebook.com/CoCreativeSex
cocreativesex.com/programs/

REFERENCES

Sexual abuse. American Psychological Association.
https://www.apa.org/topics/sexual-abuse/

UN Action Against Sexual Violence in Conflict, http://www.stoprapenow.org/news/

Sexual Violence: a Tool of War, Outreach Programme on the Rwanda Genocide and the United Nations. (2014) https://www.un.org/en/preventgenocide/rwanda/assets/pdf/Backgrounder%20Sexual%20Violence%202014.pdf

Post-Traumatic Stress Disorder, Canadian Mental Health Association, https://toronto.cmha.ca/documents/post-traumatic-stress-disorder-ptsd/

Paterson, Kerry. *(2016, July 13) When Rape Became a War Crime (hint: It's not when you think).* http://www.womensmediacenter.com/women-under-siege/when-rape-became-a-war-crime-hint-its-not-when-you-think1

Barmark, Sarah. *(2018, Jan. 18) What Consent Means in the Age of #MeToo.* https://thewalrus.ca/what-consent-means-in-the-age-of-metoo/

References

Levenson, Eric and Aaron Cooper. (2018, April 26) Bill Cosby Guilty on All Three Counts in Indecent Assault Trial. https://www.cnn.com/2018/04/26/us/bill-cosby-trial/index.html

Harvey Weinstein Charged with Rape Following New York Arrest. (2018, May 25) https://www.bbc.com/news/world-us-canada-44257202

Children and Teens: Statistics, RAINN. https://www.rainn.org/statistics/children-and-teens

Affirmative Consent Laws (Yes Means Yes) State by State. http://affirmativeconsent.com/affirmative-consent-laws-state-by-state/

Goldsworthy, Terry. (2018, Jan. 29) Yes Means Yes: Moving to a Different Model of Consent for Sexual Interactions. http://theconversation.com/yes-means-yes-moving-to-a-different-model-of-consent-for-sexual-interactions-90630

Farley, Melissa, Nicole Matthews, Sarah Deer, Guadalupe Lopez, Christine Start, Eileen Hudon. (2011. Oct. 27) Garden of Truth: The Prostitution and Trafficking of Native Women in Minnesota. A project of Minnesota Indian Women's Sexual Assault Coalition and Prostitution Research & Education. http://www.prostitutionresearch.com/pdfs/Garden_of_Truth_Final_Project_WEB.pdf

Reuniting: Healing with Sexual Relationships. www.reuniting.info

Walters, Alexander. (2014, May 12) Internet Porn Ruined My Life. http://www.vice.com/read/internet-porn-ruined-my-life

Bolton, Doug. (2015, May 10) Porn And Video Game Addiction Leading to 'Masculinity Crisis,' Says Stanford Psychologist. https://www.independent.co.uk/news/science/porn-and-video-game-addiction-are-leading-to-masculinity-crisis-says-stanford-prison-experiment-10238211.html

Worstall, Tim. (2012, June 8) The Declining Economics of the Pornography Industry. https://www.forbes.com/sites/tim-worstall/2012/06/08/the-declining-economics-of-the-pornography-industry/#7a81447d7fa7

Dines, Gail and Dana Bialer. (2012. June 7) Porn is in Rude Health, The Guardian. https://www.theguardian.com/commentisfree/2012/jun/07/porn-rude-health-louis-theroux

Pathological Gambling Changes in the DSM-5. (2012. June 1) Responsible Gambling Council. https://www.responsiblegambling.org/rg-news-research/newscan/newscan-item/2012/06/01/pathological-gambling-changes-in-the-dsm-5

What is Gambling Disorder. The American Psychiatric Association. (https://www.psychiatry.org/patients-families/gambling-disorder/what-is-gambling-disorder

Weir, Kirsten. (2014, April) Is Pornography Addictive? American Psychological Association. https://www.apa.org/monitor/2014/04/pornography

Levin, Sam. (2017, Jan. 25) 'End of an Era': Porn Actors Lament the Loss of Legendary San Francisco Armory. https://www.theguardian.com/culture/2017/jan/25/porn-bdsm-kink-armory-closing-san-francisco

References

Michelwait, Laila. (2017, Jan 27) World's Largest Torture Porn Studio Shuts Its Doors, Exodus Cry. https://exoduscry.com/blog/general/worlds-largest-torture-porn-studio-shuts-doors/

Auerbach, David. (2014, Oct 23) Vampire Porn: MindGeek is a cautionary tale of consolidating production and distribution in a single, monopolistic owner, Slate. https://slate.com/technology/2014/10/mindgeek-porn-monopoly-its-dominance-is-a-cautionary-tale-for-other-industries.html

Tolentino, Jia. (2018, May 15) The Rage of the Incels, The New Yorker. https://www.newyorker.com/culture/cultural-comment/the-rage-of-the-incels

Pinsker, Joe. (2016, Apr 4) The Hidden Economics of Porn. https://www.theatlantic.com/business/archive/2016/04/pornography-industry-economics-tarrant/476580/

Ashley Voss, Hilarie Cash, Sean Hurdiss, Frank Bishop, Warren P. Klam, and Andrew P. Doan, (2015, Sept) Case Report: Internet Gaming Disorder Associated With Pornography Use, Yale J Biol Med.; 88(3): 319–324. https://www.ncbi.nlm.nih.gov/pmc/articles/PMC4553653/#R17

Doidge, Norman. (2007, December 18) The Brain That Changes Itself: Stories of Personal Triumph from the Frontiers of Brain Science, Penguin Books

Love, Todd, & all. (2015, Sept) Neuroscience of Internet Pornography Addiction: A Review and Update, Behavior Science (Basel). 5(3): 388–433. https://www.ncbi.nlm.nih.gov/pmc/articles/PMC4600144/

Hilton, Donald L. Jr. (2013, Jul 19) Pornography Addiction - A Supranormal Stimulus Considered in the Context of Neuroplasticity. Socioaffect Neuroscience Psychology.19;3:20767. doi: 10.3402/snp. v3i0.20767. eCollection 2013

Keach, Sean. (2018, April 18) Fortnite Players Flood onto Pornhub in Search Of XXX Game Clips As Game Goes Offline. https://www.news.com.au/technology/home-entertainment/gaming/fortnite-players-flood-onto-pornhub-in-search-of-xxx-game-clips-as-game-goes-offline/news-story/351daf6c5d28d19c3a7c3d51335586b8

Brenton, Hannah. (2018, March 23) MindGeek: Porn empire reports half billion dollars in revenue—but ends year with loss, Luxembourg Times. https://luxtimes.lu/luxembourg/33248-porn-empire-reports-half-billion-dollars-in-revenue-but-ends-year-with-loss

Richtel, Matt. (2013, Sept. 21) Intimacy on the Web, With a Crowd, The New York Times. https://www.nytimes.com/2013/09/22/technology/intimacy-on-the-web-with-a-crowd.html

de Alarcón, Ruben & al. (2019, Jan. 15) J. Clin. Med. 2019, Online Porn Addiction: What We Know and What We Don't—A Systematic Review, J. Clin. Med. 2019, 8(1), 91; doi: 10.3390/jcm8010091

https://www.mdpi.com/2077-0383/8/1/91

Brand, M. & al. (2014, May 27) Prefrontal Control and Internet Addiction: A Theoretical Model and Review of Neuropsychological and Neuroimaging Findings. Front Hum Neurosci. 2014 May 27;8:375. https://www.ncbi.nlm.nih.gov/pubmed/24904393#

References

Chen KH. & al. (2018, July 12) *Internet Gaming Disorder: An Emergent Health Issue for Men. Am J Mens Health.* 12(4):1151-1159. doi: 10.1177/1557988318766950. Epub 2018 Apr 1. https://www.ncbi.nlm.nih.gov/pubmed/29606034#

Peters, Sarah. (2013, December) *Youth and Pornography Addiction, the Fix: Addiction and Recovery, Straight Up.* https://www.thefix.com/content/youth-and-pornography-addiction

Griggs, Brandon. (2016, Feb. 24) *Terry Crew: Porn Addiction Messed up My Life.* https://www.cnn.com/2016/02/24/entertainment/terry-crews-porn-addition-feat/index.html

Hayes, Mark. (2014, April 15) https://www.irishexaminer.com/lifestyle/features/why-porn-is-finally-going-down-the-tube-265332.html

Julian, Kate. (2018, Dec.) *"Why Are Young People Having So Little Sex," The Atlantic.* https://www.theatlantic.com/magazine/archive/2018/12/the-sex-recession/573949/

Davies, Jack. (2013, Dec. 9) *I Spent a Month Living in a Romanian Sexcam Studio, Vice.* https://www.vice.com/en_us/article/mv5e3n/bucharest-webcam-studios-america-outsourcing-sex-trade

Bui, Thao-Mi. (2017, Sept. 15) *The Economics of Pornography Stripped Down.* http://economicstudents.com/2017/09/economics-pornography-stripped/#_ftn3

Biddle, Sam. (2012, Sept 18) https://gizmodo.com/5941976/indentured-servitude-money-laundering-and-piles-of-money-the-crazy-secrets-of-internet-cam-girls-nsfw

Dunne, Sean. (2016) *Cam Girlz, veryape.tv.* https://vimeo.com/155155963,

Porn-o-nomics: Why a Multi-Billion-Dollar Industry is Having So Much Trouble Actually Making Money. (2017, Feb. 10) CBC. https://www.cbc.ca/amp/1.3972917

How Does the Porn Industry Actually Make Money? (2018, June) Fight the New Drug. https://fightthenewdrug.org/how-does-the-porn-industry-actually-make-money-today/

Porn Is a 12 billion Industry but Profits Leave the Valley. (2017, August 29) Daily News. https://www.dailynews.com/2007/06/05/porn-is-a-12-billion-industry-but-profits-leave-the-valley/

How the Porn Business Works, What it Makes, and What its Future May Be, PBS. (https://www.pbs.org/wgbh/pages/frontline/shows/porn/business/howtheme.html

Ackman, Dan. (2001, May 25) *How Big is Porn? Forbes.* https://www.forbes.com/2001/05/25/0524porn.html#291c30179845

Silver, Curtis. (2018, Jan 9) *Pornhub 2017 Year In Review Insights Report Reveals Statistical Proof We Love Porn, Forbes.* https://www.forbes.com/sites/curtissilver/2018/01/09/pornhub-2017-year-in-review-insights-report-reveals-statistical-proof-we-love-porn/#46e7636624f5

Borreli, Lizette. (2016, Sept. 7) *Sexual Facts About Women: What Are Multiple Orgasms And How To Achieve The 'Double O,' Medical Daily.* https://www.medicaldaily.com/sexual-facts-about-women-what-are-multiple-orgasms-and-how-achieve-double-o-397190

References

Thomshauer, Regena. (2016 September) Pussy: A Reclamation. Hay House

Hardy, Janet W. and Dossie Easton. (1997, 2009, 2017) The Ethical Slut, 3rd ed., Ten Speed Press

Nagoski, Emily. (2015, March) Come As You Are. Simon & Schuster Paperbacks

Chia, Mantak, Maneewan Chia, Douglas Abrams & Rachel Carlton Abrams. (2000) The Multi-Orgasmic Couple. Harper One

Deida, David. (1997, 2004) The Way of the Superior Man, 2nd Ed. Sounds True, Boulder.

Pailet, Xanet. (2018) Living an Orgasmic Life. Mango Publishing

Deida, David. (1995) Intimate Communion. Health Communication Inc.

Dispenza, Joe. (2017, 2019) Becoming Supernatural. Hay House, Inc.

Ward, Devi. (2012) Shake Your Soul Song! Dakini Dancer Press

Rilke, Rainer Maria. (1975) Rilke on Love and Other Difficulties, Translations and considerations by John J.L. Mood, W.W. Norton & Company, Inc.

Miller, Alice. (2006) The Body Never Lies, W.W. Norton & Company, Inc.

Beras, Erika. (2017, April 15) *Traces of Genetic Trauma Can Be Tweaked, Scientific American.* https://www.scientificamerican.com/podcast/episode/traces-of-genetic-trauma-can-be-tweaked/

Dale, Cyndi. (2011) *Energetic Boundaries: How to Stay Connected in Work, Love, and Life,* Sounds True, Boulder

Pierrakos, Eva and Judith Saly. (1993, 2002) *Creating Union: The Essence of Intimate Relationships,* Second Edition, Pathwork Press

Women Writing Culture (1995) Ed. by Ruth Behar and Deborah A. Gordon, University of California Press

Favor Hamilton, Suzy. (2015) *Fast Girl: A Life Spent Running from Madness,* Harper Collins

Bonheim, Jalaha. (1997) *Aphrodite's Daughters: Women's Sexual Stories and the Journey of the Soul,* Simon & Schuster

Hagel, Caia and Tatiana Fraser. (2016) *Girl Positive: Supporting Girls to Shape a New World,* Penguin Random House, 2016

Moran, Rachel. (2015) *Paid For: My Journey Through Prostitution,* W.W. Norton & Company, Inc.

Blacklege, Catherine. (2014) *The Story of V: A Natural History of Female Sexuality,* Rutgers University Press, 2004

Perel, Esther. (2006) *Mating in Captivity.* Harper Collins

ACKNOWLEDGMENTS

Thank you Diana Dorell, Laura Bailey, Jenny McKaig, Maria Palumbo, Catherine Mellon, Catherine Dubreuil and Friesen Press for advising me and editing my book.

Thank you Mom, Dad, James, Beth, Geoff, Epiphany, Shawn, Matt, Sky, Devi, Baljit, Josée, Dulani, Jason, Peter, Sarah, Michel M., Patrick M. for giving me feedback and/or significant support along the way.

Thank you Geoff Affleck and Janette Anderson for helping me birth the title!

Thank you to ALL these wonderful thought and transformational leaders that have been tremendously inspiring along this book writing journey! Thank you Baljit Rayat for believing in me and holding space for me from the very inception—until completion.